Copyright

Copyright © 2024 by Dr. Kama Kamzy

All rights reserved. No part of this publication may be reproduced, distributed, or transmitted in any form or by any means, including photocopying, recording, or other electronic or mechanical methods, without the prior written permission of the publisher, except in the case of brief quotations embodied in critical reviews and certain other noncommercial uses permitted by copyright law.

Disclaimer

The information provided in this book is for educational and informational purposes only and is not intended as medical advice. It is not a substitute for professional medical advice, diagnosis, or treatment. Always seek the advice of your physician or other qualified health provider with any questions you may have regarding a medical condition.

The author and publisher of this book are not liable for any loss, injury, or damage incurred as a result of the use of the information provided in this book. The reader assumes full responsibility for consulting a qualified healthcare professional regarding health conditions and concerns, and for any decisions made or actions taken based on the information contained in this book.

The views expressed in this book are those of the author and do not necessarily reflect the views of the publisher. The author has made every effort to ensure the accuracy and completeness of the information presented, but cannot guarantee that the information is free from errors or omissions.

The inclusion of specific products, services, or resources in this book does not imply endorsement by the author or publisher. It is the responsibility of the reader to evaluate the suitability of any product, service, or resource mentioned in this book for their own use.

By reading this book, you acknowledge and agree to the terms of this disclaimer. If you do not agree with these terms, you should not use the information provided in this book.

Thank you for your understanding and cooperation.

Sincerely,

Dr. Kama Kamzy

Here's Your BONUS!
A 30-Day Meal Plan

DAY 1

- Breakfast: Spinach & Egg Scramble with Raspberries
- Lunch: Mason Jar Power Salad with Chickpeas & Tuna
- Dinner: Grilled Salmon with Sweet Peppers

DAY 2

- Breakfast: Muesli with Raspberries
- Lunch: Brussels Sprouts Salad with Crunchy Chickpeas
- Dinner: Herb-Grilled Chicken Frites

Day 3

- Breakfast: Muffin-Tin Omelets with Feta & Peppers
- Lunch: Grilled Eggplant & Tomato Pasta
- Dinner: Muesli with Raspberries

Day 4

- Breakfast: Brussels Sprouts Salad with Crunchy Chickpeas
- Lunch: Grilled Chicken Tacos with Slaw & Lime Crema
- Dinner: Guacamole Chopped Salad
- Dinner: Chicken Caesar Pasta Salad

Day 5

- Breakfast: Muffin-Tin Omelets with Feta & Peppers
- Lunch: Brussels Sprouts Salad with Crunchy Chickpeas

Day 6

- Breakfast: Muesli with Raspberries

- Lunch: Chicken Caesar Pasta Salad
- Dinner: Spring Green Frittata

Day 7

- Breakfast: Spinach & Egg Scramble with Raspberries
- Lunch: Chicken Caesar Pasta Salad
- Dinner: Greek Salad with Edamame

Day 8

- Breakfast: White Bean & Avocado Toast
- Lunch: Superfood Chopped Salad with Salmon & Creamy Garlic Dressing
- Dinner: Spinach, Peanut Butter & Banana Smoothie

Day 9

- Breakfast: Spicy Slaw Bowls with Shrimp & Edamame
- Lunch: Chicken & Veggie Fajitas
- Dinner: Grilled Flank Steak with Tomato Salad

Day 10

- Breakfast: One-Pot Chicken Pesto Pasta with Asparagus
- Lunch: Better-Than-Takeout Burgers with Sweet Potato Fries
- Dinner: Chicken & Veggie Fajitas

Day 11

- Breakfast: Spinach & Egg Scramble with Raspberries
- Lunch: Mason Jar Power Salad with Chickpeas & Tuna
- Dinner: Grilled Salmon with Sweet Peppers

Day 12

- Breakfast: Muesli with Raspberries
- Lunch: Brussels Sprouts Salad with Crunchy Chickpeas
- Dinner: Herb-Grilled Chicken Frites

Day 13

- Breakfast: Muffin-Tin Omelets with Feta & Peppers
- Lunch: Grilled Eggplant & Tomato Pasta
- Dinner: Muesli with Raspberries

Day 14

- Breakfast: Brussels Sprouts Salad with Crunchy Chickpeas
- Lunch: Grilled Chicken Tacos with Slaw & Lime Crema
- Dinner: Guacamole Chopped Salad

Day 15
- Breakfast: Muffin-Tin Omelets with Feta & Peppers
- Lunch: Brussels Sprouts Salad with Crunchy Chickpeas
- Dinner: Chicken Caesar Pasta Salad

Day 16
Breakfast: Muesli with Raspberries

Lunch: Chicken Caesar Pasta Salad

Dinner: Spring Green Frittata

Day 17
- Breakfast: Spinach & Egg Scramble with Raspberries
- Lunch: Chicken Caesar Pasta Salad
- Dinner: Greek Salad with Edamame

Day 18
- Breakfast: White Bean & Avocado Toast
- Lunch: Superfood Chopped Salad with Salmon & Creamy Garlic Dressing
- Dinner: Spinach, Peanut Butter & Banana Smoothie

Day 19
- Breakfast: Spicy Slaw Bowls with Shrimp & Edamame
- Lunch: Chicken & Veggie Fajitas
- Dinner: Grilled Flank Steak with Tomato Salad

Day 20
- Breakfast: One-Pot Chicken Pesto Pasta with Asparagus
- Lunch: Better-Than-Takeout Burgers with Sweet Potato Fries
- Dinner: Spicy Slaw Bowls with Shrimp & Edamame

Day 21
- Breakfast: Spinach & Egg Scramble with Raspberries
- Lunch: Mason Jar Power Salad with Chickpeas & Tuna
- Dinner: Grilled Salmon with Sweet Peppers

Day 22
- Breakfast: Muesli with Raspberries
- Lunch: Brussels Sprouts Salad with Crunchy Chickpeas
- Dinner: Herb-Grilled Chicken Frites

Day 23
- Breakfast: Muffin-Tin Omelets with Feta & Peppers
- Lunch: Grilled Eggplant & Tomato Pasta
- Dinner: Muesli with Raspberries

Day 24
- Breakfast: Brussels Sprouts Salad with Crunchy Chickpeas
- Lunch: Grilled Chicken Tacos with Slaw & Lime Crema
- Dinner: Guacamole Chopped Salad

Day 25
- Breakfast: Muffin-Tin Omelets with Feta & Peppers
- Lunch: Brussels Sprouts Salad with Crunchy Chickpeas
- Dinner: Chicken Caesar Pasta Salad

Day 26
- Breakfast: Muesli with Raspberries
- Lunch: Chicken Caesar Pasta Salad
- Dinner: Spring Green Frittata

Day 27
- Breakfast: Spinach & Egg Scramble with Raspberries
- Lunch: Chicken Caesar Pasta Salad
- Dinner: Greek Salad with Edamame

Day 28
- Breakfast: White Bean & Avocado Toast
- Lunch: Superfood Chopped Salad with Salmon & Creamy Garlic Dressing
- Dinner: Spinach, Peanut Butter & Banana Smoothie

Day 29
- Breakfast: Spicy Slaw Bowls with Shrimp & Edamame
- Lunch: Chicken & Veggie Fajitas
- Dinner: Grilled Flank Steak with Tomato Salad

Day 30
- Breakfast: One-Pot Chicken Pesto Pasta with Asparagus
- Lunch: Better-Than-Takeout Burgers with Sweet Potato Fries
- Dinner: Spicy Slaw Bowls with Shrimp & Edamame

About the Author

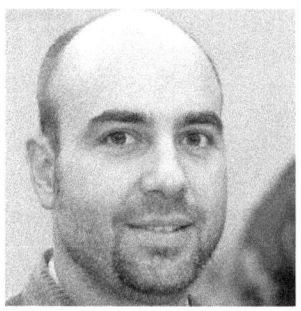

Dr. Kama Kamzy is a passionate advocate for healthy living and lifestyle. With a background in medicine, Dr. Kamzy has dedicated his career to promoting holistic approaches to health and well-being. His expertise in the medical field, coupled with his personal interest in healthy living, has led him to explore various aspects of wellness, including nutrition, fitness, and mindful living.

Dr. Kamzy believes in the power of preventive medicine and the importance of lifestyle choices in maintaining optimal health. Through his work, he aims to educate and empower individuals to make informed decisions about their health, emphasizing the role of nutrition, exercise, and stress management in achieving overall wellness.

In addition to his professional pursuits, Dr. Kamzy is a devoted husband and family man. He understands the challenges of balancing a busy career with personal life and strives to integrate his passion for health into his everyday routine. His commitment to leading by example and practicing what he preaches is evident in his own lifestyle choices and the values he instills in his family.

Dr. Kamzy's holistic approach to health and wellness is reflected in his writing, where he combines his medical expertise with practical advice and insights to inspire others to live healthier, happier lives. He is dedicated to sharing his knowledge and experiences to help individuals achieve their health goals and lead fulfilling lives.

You can connect with Dr. Kama Kamzy and stay updated on his latest work by following him on https://www.amazon.com/author/drkamakamzy.com. Thank you for joining him on this journey towards better health and well-being.

Warm regards,

Dr. Kama Kamzy

Table of Contents:

Copyright 4
Disclaimer 6
Here's Your BONUS! 7
About the Author 11
Table of Contents: 13
Introduction 17
    Brief History of Somatic Exercises 17
    What are Somatic Exercises 17
    Understanding the Mind-Body Connection 17
    How Somatic Exercises Aid in Weight Loss 18
    Importance of Consistency and Mindfulness 18
Chapter 1: 19
Getting Started! 19
How to Use This Book 19
    Setting Realistic Goals 20
    Creating a Supportive Environment 21
Chapter 2: 23
Benefits of Somatic Exercises 23
    1. Improved posture and body awareness 24
    2. Stress Reduction and Relaxation 24
    3.   Enhanced Flexibility and Range of Motion 24
    4.   Alleviation of Chronic Pain and Tension 24
    5. Help with Weight Loss and Healthy Living 24
Chapter 3: 25
Warm-Up Somatic Exercises 25
    Purpose of Warm-Up Somatic Exercises 25
    Benefits of Warm-Up Somatic Exercises 25
Chapter 4: 29
Beginners Level Somatic Exercises 29
    Benefits of Beginner Level Somatic Exercises 30
    Basic Movements for Those New to Somatics 30

    Building Awareness of Muscle Tension 32

    Techniques for Building Awareness of Muscle Tension.. 32

    Tools to Relieve Tension 33

Chapter 5: 35

Intermediate Level Somatic Exercises 35

    Progressing to More Complex Movements 35

    Deepening Body Awareness and Control 35

    Integrating Somatics into Daily Life 36

    What Makes Intermediate Somatic Exercises Different?... 36

Chapter 6: Advanced Level Somatic Exercises... 41

    Challenging the Body with Advanced Sequences 41

    Fine-Tuning Movement Patterns 41

    Incorporating Somatics into Fitness Routines 41

    What Sets Advanced Somatic Exercises Apart?... 41

    Are you ready to ascend? Example of Advanced Somatic Exercises: 42

Chapter 7: 30-Day Somatic Exercise Routine... 46

Day 1:	Diaphragmatic Breathing	TIME: 30 MINUTES	46
Day 2:	Grounding	TIME: 25 MINUTES	46
Day 3:	Body Scanning	TIME: 15 MINUTES	47
Day 5:	Breathwork & Arm Circles	TIME: 15 MINUTES	50
Day 6:	Pelvic Tilts & Spinal Waves	TIME: 15 MINUTES	51
Day 7:	Rest & Reflection (Free Day)	TIME: HOURS	52
Day 8:	SENSORY AWARENESS	TIME: 30 MINUTES	53
Day 9:	The Voo Breath	TIME: 15 MINUTES	54
Day 10:	Self-Hug	TIME: 15 MINUTES	55
Day 11:	Eagle Poses	TIME: 15 MINUTES	56
Day 12:	Superman	TIME: 20 MINUTES	58
Day 13:	Knee Hold	TIME: 15 MINUTES	60
Day 14:	Rest & Reflection (Free Day)	TIME: HOURS	61
Day 15:	Jumping Jacks	TIME: 25 MINUTES	62
Day 16:	Reach Back	TIME: 25 MINUTES	63
Day 17:	Body Rocking	TIME: 30 MINUTES	64

Day 18:	Side Reach	TIME: 30 MINUTES	65
Day 19:	Hip Circles	TIME: 30 MINUTES	67
Day 20:	Spinal Rotations	TIME: 30 MINUTES	68
Day 21:	Rest & Reflection (Free Day)	TIME: HOURS	69
Day 22:	Arm Swings	TIME: 30 MINUTES	70
Day 23:	Leg Pendulum	TIME: 25 MINUTES	71
Day 24:	Hip and Pelvic Stability	TIME: 25 MINUTES	72
Day 25:	Mindful Walking	TIME: 30 MINUTES	73
Day 26:	Lower Body Awareness	TIME: 30 MINUTES	74
Day 27:	Modified Burpees	TIME: 30 MINUTES	76
Day 28:	Rest & Reflection	TIME: 60 MINUTES	78
Day 29:	Chest Opening	TIME: 30 MINUTES	79
Day 30:	Baby Stretch	TIME: 30 MINUTES	81

Chapter 8: Somatic Workouts 82
   Benefits of Somatic Workout 83
   Sample Somatic Workout Routine 84
   Integrating Somatics into Traditional Workouts 84
   Advantages of Integrating Somatics: 85
   Creating Balanced Fitness Programs 86
   Principles for Developing a Balanced Fitness Program 87

Chapter 9: 30-Day Weight Loss Smoothies 90
   Blackberry Smoothie 90
   Strawberry-Banana Protein Smoothie 91
   Banana-Cocoa Soy Smoothie 93
   Anti-Inflammatory Beet Smoothie 94
   Cherry-Berry Oatmeal Smoothies 95
   Strawberry-Chocolate Smoothie 96
   Ultimate Healthy Breakfast Smoothie 97
   Chocolate-Banana Protein Smoothie 98
   Grape Smoothie 99
   Pineapple Green Smoothie 100
   Strawberry-Blueberry-Banana Smoothie 101

Fruit & Yogurt Smoothie 102
Spinach-Avocado Smoothie 103
Carrot-Apple Smoothie 104
Passion Fruit Smoothie 105
Cherry-Mocha Smoothie 106
Berry-Kefir Smoothie 107
Avocado & Banana Smoothie 108
Strawberry-Mango-Banana Smoothie 109
Thermos-Ready Smoothie 110
Creamsicle Breakfast Smoothie 111
Berry-Coconut Smoothie 112
Pumpkin Pie Smoothie 113
Peanut Butter-Strawberry-Kale Smoothie 114
Mango-Ginger Smoothie 115
Blueberry-Cranberry Smoothie 116
Cantaloupe Smoothie 117
Strawberry-Pineapple Smoothie 118
Jason Mraz's Avocado Green Smoothie 119
Mango Raspberry Smoothie 120
Recipes for Nutrient-Dense Smoothies 121
Incorporating Somatic Principles into Nutrition 123
Supporting Weight Loss with Healthy Eating 124

Conclusion 128
Recap of Key Points: 128
Motivation for Long-Term Success: 128

I Have a Request 130

ADDITIONAL RESOURCES 131

Introduction

In recent years, there has been a surge of interest in holistic approaches to health and wellness, with an emphasis on the interdependence of the mind and body. Somatic exercises, based on a thorough understanding of the mind-body link, have emerged as an effective technique for not only relieving chronic pain and stress, but also promoting weight reduction and overall well-being.

Brief History of Somatic Exercises

Somatic exercises originated with the pioneering work of Thomas Hanna approach in 1990, a philosopher and movement therapist. Hanna founded the science of somatic on the assumption that our bodies contain patterns of muscle tension and movement habits that can be learnt and unlearned via concentrated awareness and motion.

Somatic education strives to retrain the nervous system and restore muscle and joint function to its optimal level. The first third of the session finished just days before Tom died in a vehicle accident. Two members of that class were principally responsible for developing the Somatic Systems Institute curriculum.

What are Somatic Exercises

Recently, the term "somatic" has been utilized extensively. There are several fields that have modified the term to describe anything that involves both the mind and the body, and they are somewhat right. In reality, somatic comes from the word soma, which Dr. Hanna used to characterize the full and indivisible essence of the human being. This means that rather than working with the mind and body, there is an implicit understanding that each person is the mind and body combined--a holistic and global understanding of the biological, cultural, emotional, psychological, spiritual, energetic, and evolutionary functioning of the human organism.

Somatic exercises are a series of gentle movements designed to reprogram the brain's control of muscles, promoting relaxation and improved movement patterns. Unlike traditional exercise programs that focus solely on physical exertion, somatic exercises emphasize the internal experience of movement, encouraging practitioners to develop a heightened awareness of their body's sensations and responses.

Understanding the Mind-Body Connection

Recognizing the complex interaction between mind and body is central to somatic exercise practice. Muscular tension and pain are physical manifestations of stress, anxiety, and emotional trauma. Somatic exercises offer a method to release these stored tensions, providing a sensation of relaxation and well-being in both the body and mind.

How Somatic Exercises Aid in Weight Loss

When it comes to weight loss, somatic exercises provide a novel method that goes beyond traditional diet and exercise plans. Somatic exercises can help people build a more conscious and intuitive relationship with their bodies by addressing the underlying patterns of tension and stress that contribute to harmful behaviors and emotional eating, resulting in long-term weight loss and healthier body composition.

Importance of Consistency and Mindfulness

Like any form of exercise or therapy, consistency is key to reaping the benefits of somatic exercises. By practicing regularly and with mindful awareness, individuals can gradually release chronic patterns of tension, improve their posture and movement, and cultivate a deeper connection with their bodies. This book is designed to guide you through the principles and practices of somatic exercises, offering a comprehensive approach to achieving your weight loss goals while nurturing a greater sense of well-being.

Chapter 1:

Getting Started!

How to Use This Book

This book is intended to be a complete guide on incorporating somatic exercises into your life to help you lose weight and improve your general well-being. Whether you're new to somatic exercises or have some experience, this chapter will show you how to get the most out of this book.

1. Understanding the structure

The book is divided into several chapters, each focusing on different aspects of somatic exercises and their application to weight loss. It begins with an overview of somatic exercises, their history, and advantages. The next chapters include warm-up exercises, beginning, middle, and advanced level exercises, 30-day routines, workouts, and weight loss smoothies.

2. Set Your Goals

Before you begin the workouts, consider your own goals. Are you primarily want to lose weight, improve your posture, or relieve muscular tension? Setting specific objectives can help you maintain focus and motivation throughout your somatic journey.

3. Navigating the Exercises

Each chapter includes thorough exercise instructions, graphics, and links to video demonstrations. Warm-up exercises should be performed first to prepare your body for the more difficult actions that come next. As you go through the book, you will encounter exercises designed to various levels of expertise, ranging from beginners to advanced practitioners.

4. Setting Your Routine

To get the most out of this book, consider developing a daily or weekly regimen that includes somatic exercises. Consistency is essential, so attempt to practice on a regular basis, even if it's only for a few minutes every day. You can follow the 30-day routines outlined in the book or create your own based on your tastes and schedule.

5. Tracking your progress

Keeping track of your progress may be quite motivating. Consider keeping a record of your experiences with somatic exercises, documenting any changes in your body, emotions, or overall health. You may also wish to monitor your weight, measurements, or other relevant metrics to determine the effectiveness of the activities.

Setting Realistic Goals

Before beginning any new fitness or health journey, it is critical to establish reasonable and attainable goals. This is especially true when it comes to somatic exercises for weight reduction, as the process entails more than simply physical movements—it also a mental change and a dedication to long-term health. Here are some suggestions for developing realistic goals:

1. **Be specific**

   Instead of making a general goal like "lose weight," be precise about what you want to accomplish. For example, you may establish a goal like "lose 10 pounds in three months" or "improve my posture and reduce back pain."

2. **Make them Measurable.**

   Goals should be quantifiable so that you can monitor your progress. This may include recording your weight, collecting body measurements, or maintaining a log of how you feel after doing somatic exercises.

3. **Establish a Timeline**

   Give yourself a realistic timetable for achieving your goals. Avoid establishing unreasonable deadlines, which may lead to disappointment or exhaustion. Instead, concentrate on making steady growth over time.

4. **Evaluate Your Lifestyle**

   When making objectives, remember to consider your present lifestyle and obligations. If you have a hectic schedule, be realistic about the amount of time you can devote to somatic exercises each day.

5. **Be Flexible**

   While it's essential to have goals, it's also important to be flexible and adaptable. Life can be unpredictable, and you may need to adjust your goals or timeline along the way. This doesn't mean giving up on your goals; it means being realistic and kind to yourself as you navigate your journey.

Setting reasonable and achievable objectives for your somatic exercise practice can keep you motivated and focused on your journey to better health and weight loss. Remember that growth is not always linear, and it is acceptable to make tiny steps as long as you are going ahead.

Creating a Supportive Environment

Starting a somatic exercise journey for weight reduction demands more than just physical effort; it also entails developing a supportive atmosphere that promotes your objectives and well-being. Here are some suggestions for establishing a supportive setting for your somatic exercise practice.

1. **Clear Space for Practice**

    Designate a calm, clutter-free area in your house where you may practice your somatic exercises without interruption. Having a specific place can help you focus and immerse yourself in the exercise.

2. **Gather the Right Tools**

    While somatic exercises are largely focused on your body and mind, having the correct equipment can help you improve your practice. This might include a yoga mat or comfy attire that allows for freedom of movement. Consider any additional tools or accessories that may be useful in your practice, such as a cushion for sitting meditation or a small stool for balancing exercises.

3. **Seek Support from Others**

    Consider sharing your somatic exercise adventure with friends, family, or a support group. A support system may give encouragement, accountability, and inspiration on days when you feel unmotivated.

4. **Practice Mindfulness in Your Daily Life**

    Somatic exercises are more than just time spent on the mat; they can be incorporated into your everyday routine. Pay attention to your body's feelings and movements whether walking, sitting, or eating.

5. **Prioritize Self-Care.**

    Incorporate self-care activities into your daily routine to aid in your somatic exercise journey. This might involve things like meditation, deep breathing exercises, or simply taking time to relax and rejuvenate.

Chapter 2:

Benefits of Somatic Exercises

A woman lived in a crowded city and had struggled with weight control for years. Despite attempting several diets and exercise regimes, she struggled to obtain lasting results. She was dissatisfied and dismayed when she came across somatic exercises while investigating holistic weight loss methods. She was intrigued by the concept of treating both the physical and emotional components of weight control and decided to try somatic workouts. She began with simple warm-up exercises and eventually progressed to attentive movements, focusing on her body's feelings. As she went through the basic and intermediate levels, she noticed small differences in her body's flexibility and overall sense of well-being. Motivated by these early good results, she committed to regular practice and included advanced routines into her program. With each session, she grew more aware of her body and learned to move with elegance and focus. Over time, she not only lost weight but also improved her posture, energy levels, and general confidence.

Her somatic exercise adventure helped her get a better awareness of her body's requirements and how to nurture it with attentive movement. This increased understanding enabled her to adopt a healthy relationship with food and exercise, resulting in long-term weight loss. As she continued to practice, she felt empowered to make great choices that benefited her well-being and helped her achieve her overall weight control objectives. Today, she is appreciative for the transformational power of somatic exercises in her weight reduction journey. She not only met her weight reduction objectives but also adopted a holistic approach to health and wellbeing, allowing her to live her best life.

Somatic activities integrate the mind and body, providing a comprehensive approach to physical well-being. These exercises, which emphasize sensory-motor awareness, pandiculation, and mindful movement, have been shown to improve posture, stress levels, flexibility, and general movement patterns. Incorporating somatic exercises into one's daily routine can lead to a healthier, more balanced lifestyle, encouraging long-term well-being and a stronger connection with one's body.

Somatic exercise provides a variety of benefits that go beyond physical health. Somatic exercises, which emphasize the mind-body connection and incorporate principles of mindfulness and body awareness, can have a significant influence on many areas of your health and well-being. Here are some important advantages of doing somatic exercises:

1. Improved posture and body awareness

Somatic exercises target muscles that help people relax and build a more natural and balanced posture. This can help reduce chronic discomfort caused by improper posture.

Somatic exercises can assist you become more aware of your body and posture. By practicing gentle motions with focused attention, you may learn to release tension and improve alignment, resulting in better posture and a lower risk of musculoskeletal disorders.

2. Stress Reduction and Relaxation

The emphasis on mindful movement and sensory awareness in somatic exercises can help with stress reduction. Individuals who focus on the present moment and release muscular tension may feel more relaxed and calm.

The mindful nature of somatic exercises makes them an effective tool for reducing stress and promoting relaxation. By tuning into your body's sensations and focusing on your breath, you can calm your mind and release built-up tension, leading to a greater sense of ease and well-being.

3. Enhanced Flexibility and Range of Motion

Somatic exercises improve flexibility by relieving muscular tension and enabling a wider range of motion. This can be especially useful for people who have stiffness or restricted movement.

Regular somatic exercises can help you increase your flexibility and range of motion. You can enhance your flexibility and mobility by gently stretching and moving your body in conscious ways. This is especially useful for reducing stiffness and enhancing general comfort.

4. Alleviation of Chronic Pain and Tension

Somatic exercises are frequently utilized as a supplemental therapy to alleviate chronic pain and stress. Somatic exercises can help reduce pain and discomfort by treating the underlying source of muscle tension and encouraging relaxation, offering relief for ailments such as back pain, neck pain, and headaches.

5. Help with Weight Loss and Healthy Living

In terms of weight loss, somatic exercises provide a unique method that goes beyond typical diet and exercise plans. Somatic exercises will help you build a more attentive and intuitive relationship with your body by addressing the underlying patterns of tension and stress that contribute to harmful behaviors and emotional eating. This will assist long-term weight reduction and general health.

Chapter 3:

Warm-Up Somatic Exercises

Warm-up somatic exercises are intended to prepare your body and mind for more strenuous activity, for instance a yoga class, a dance session, or just starting your day with increased comfort and awareness. Warm-up somatic exercises are an essential part of any somatic practice. They help to prepare the body and mind for exercise, boost blood flow to the muscles, and improve general physical awareness. These soft and thoughtful movements aim to relieve tension, increase flexibility, and promote relaxation, paving the way for a more successful and pleasurable somatic exercise session.

Purpose of Warm-Up Somatic Exercises

The primary purpose of warm-up somatic exercises is to prime the body for movement while cultivating a heightened sense of body awareness. By gently engaging in these exercises, individuals can gradually transition from a state of rest or inactivity to one of readiness for more dynamic movements. This gradual approach allows for a smoother transition into more challenging exercises, reducing the risk of injury and maximizing the benefits of the practice.

Benefits of Warm-Up Somatic Exercises

Warm-up somatic exercises provide a number of advantages that improve the overall efficacy of a somatic practice, including:

- ✓ *Injury Prevention:* Somatic exercises cultivate a deeper understanding of your internal landscape, promoting better posture, coordination, and injury prevention. By gradually preparing the body for movement, warm-up exercises reduce the risk of injury by allowing the muscles and joints to adapt to increased activity gradually.
- ✓ *Improved Performance:* A proper warm-up prepares the body for more difficult activities, increasing overall performance and allowing for higher movement efficiency. By tuning into subtle sensations, you can refine your movements, making them more efficient and graceful.
- ✓ *Enhanced Body Awareness*: Warm-up exercises promote mindfulness and body awareness, helping individuals to tune into their bodies and make adjustments to their movement patterns as needed.
- ✓ *Stress Reduction:* The focused nature of warm-up somatic activities can help to induce relaxation and reduce stress, making the practice session more favorable.

Gentle exercises and breathwork can help relieve stress, leaving you feeling calmer and more focused.

Here are some examples of warm-up somatic exercises you can try:

Body Scans: Mindful body scans can be used in warm-up exercises to improve body awareness and induce calm. These scans entail mentally scanning various portions of the body, identifying any areas of tension or discomfort, and intentionally releasing them.

- Lie down comfortably on your back with your eyes closed.
- Take a few deep breaths and let your body settle into the floor.
- Begin by bringing your attention to your toes, gently wiggling them and noticing any sensations you feel.
- Slowly move your awareness up your body, paying attention to each part (feet, ankles, calves, knees, thighs, etc.) without judgment.
- As you reach your head, observe any tightness, tension, or areas that feel particularly heavy or light.
- Continue scanning your body for a few minutes, simply observing without trying to change anything.

Gentle Spinal Movements:

- Sit on the floor with your legs crossed or knees bent and grounded.
- Lengthen your spine and gently roll your neck in a small circle, forward and backward.
- Imagine your spine as a long spring, slowly making small undulations up and down.
- You can also perform gentle side bends, twisting your torso slightly while keeping your hips facing forward.
- Breathe deeply and smoothly throughout the movements.

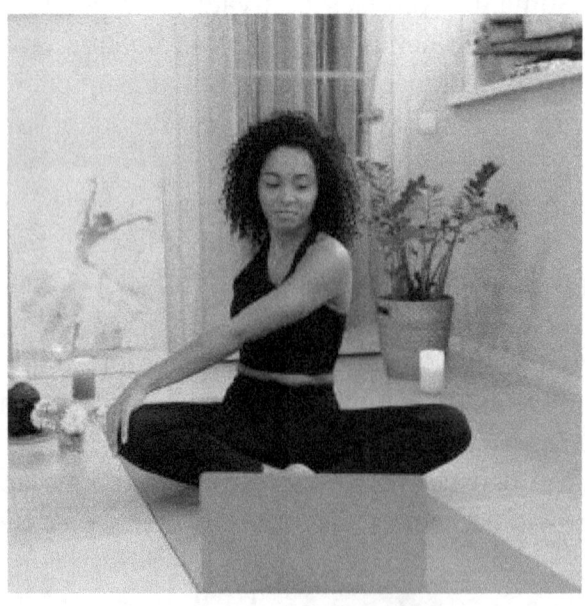

Pelvic Tilts:

- Lie on your back, knees bent, feet flat on the floor.
- Engage your core muscles by pressing your lower back into the mat and tilting your pelvis up.
- Hold for a few seconds, then slowly release. Repeat 5-10 times.
- This exercise can help relax your lower back and enhance pelvic stability.

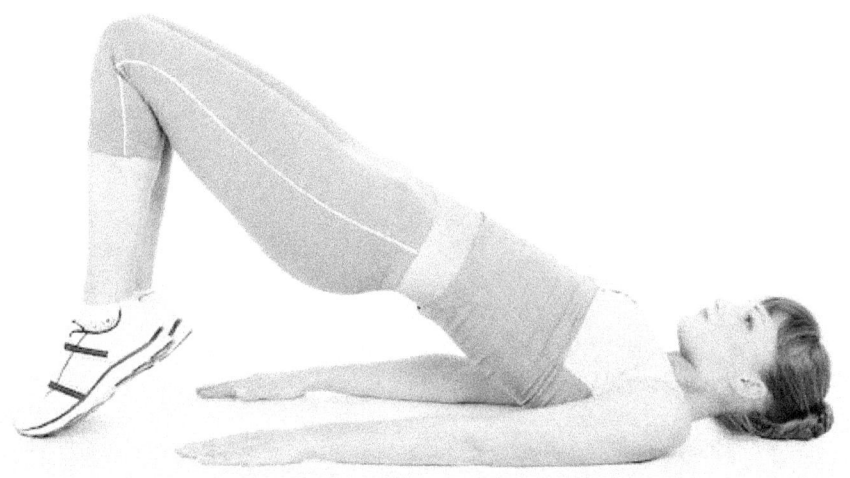

Arm Circles:

- Stand with feet hip-width apart and relaxed shoulders.
- Move your arms in tiny circles forward and backward, focusing on the sensation in your shoulder joints.
- Gradually increase the circle size and speed of movement.
- Pay attention to any areas of tightness or constriction and move lightly without exerting pressure.

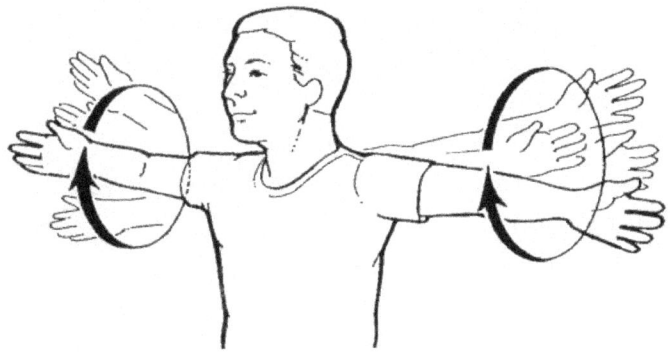

Breathing Techniques: Deep breathing exercises are frequently used in warm-up routines to center the mind, oxygenate the body, and induce relaxation. By concentrating on the breath, practitioners may build a sense of serenity and prepare the body for activity.

Breathwork;

- Sit or lie down comfortably, close your eyes.
- Put one hand on your tummy, the other on your chest.
- Inhale slowly and deeply through your nose, feeling your belly expand.
- Exhale slowly with pursed lips, feeling your belly draw in.
- Experience deep and rhythmic breathing for a few minutes, concentrating on the sensation of your breath traveling through your body.

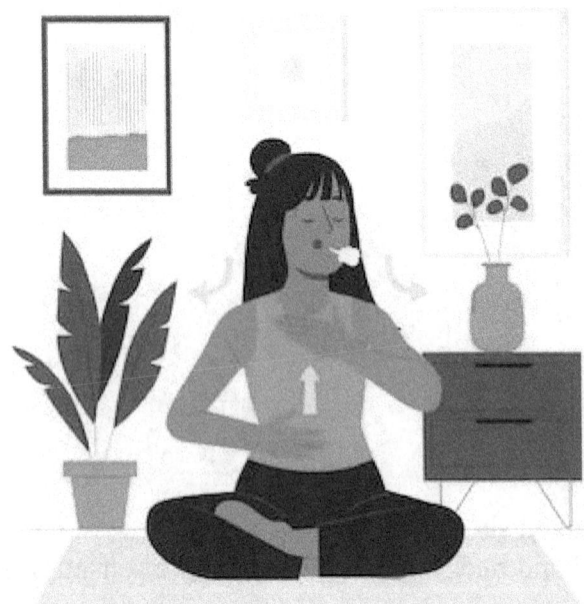

Remember:

- There are no right or incorrect ways to perform somatic exercises. Listen to your body and move in a way that feels natural and safe to you.
- Begin with modest, easy motions, then gradually raise the intensity as you grow more comfortable with the exercises.
- Focus on your breathing and let it guide your movements.
- Be patient and nice to yourself. Somatic exercises are a voyage of discovery, not a competition for perfection.

Chapter 4:

Beginners Level Somatic Exercises

In essence, beginner-level somatic exercises offer a mild introduction to somatic practice, with an emphasis on developing body awareness, relieving tension, and refining movement patterns. These exercises are suitable for people of all ages and fitness levels, and they provide a foundation for more advanced somatic activities. Beginners level somatic exercises are designed to introduce individuals to the fundamental principles and movements of somatic practice. These exercises focus on cultivating body awareness, releasing tension, and improving movement patterns in a gentle and accessible manner. They are ideal for those who are new to somatic exercises or are looking to establish a solid foundation for their practice.

Key Elements of Beginner-Level Somatic Exercises:

1. Mindful Movement: Somatic exercises for beginners focus on slow, deliberate movements that are performed with mindfulness. This method enables people to tune into their bodies, examine their usual movement patterns, and make conscious modifications as needed.

2. Breath Awareness: Breathing is an essential component of somatic exercises, and novices are advised to become aware of their breath while moving. Conscious breathing can help people relax, concentrate, and strengthen their mind-body connection.

3. Basic Muscle Contractions and Releases: Beginners learn fundamental somatic motions, such as contracting and releasing certain muscle regions. These exercises help people discover regions of tension and learn how to release habitual muscle contractions that cause pain or limited movement.

4. Exploration of Body Sensations: Beginners are taught to pay attention to areas of tension, discomfort, or ease in their bodies while performing exercises. This sensory awareness is essential for gaining a better knowledge of one's body and its movements.

5. Progressive Sequencing: Beginners' somatic exercises frequently follow progressive patterns that eventually increase in complexity. This allows people to begin with easy motions and progress as they grow more comfortable with the practice.

6. Focus on Relaxation. Beginner-level workouts often incorporate relaxation aspects to assist people release tension and stress. This emphasis on relaxation is critical for creating a conducive atmosphere for learning and performing somatic activities.

Benefits of Beginner Level Somatic Exercises

- *Improved Body Awareness*: Beginner-level somatic exercises help people become more aware of their bodies, including posture, movement patterns, and areas of stress.

- *Stress Reduction:* The focused and soothing nature of beginner-level exercises can aid in stress reduction and foster a sense of serenity and well-being.

- *Enhanced Flexibility and Mobility*: By releasing tension and refining movement patterns, novices can increase their body's flexibility and mobility.

-*Foundation for Advanced Practice*: Beginners level exercises lay the groundwork for more advanced somatic practices by introducing fundamental principles and movements.

Basic Movements for Those New to Somatics

For those new to somatic exercises, beginning with fundamental motions is critical for laying a solid foundation and developing a better knowledge of the mind-body relationship. These mild, accessible motions aim to increase body awareness, relieve tension, and improve general mobility. Here are some fundamental motions that are frequently included in beginners' somatic exercise routines:

1. Pelvic Tilts: Lie on your back, legs bent, feet flat on the floor. Gently sway your pelvis forth and backward to enable your lower back to arch and flatten. This action relieves stress in the lower back and pelvis and improves pelvic mobility. See above chapter for illustration.

2. Neck Rolls: Sit or stand comfortably, keeping your shoulders relaxed. Slowly lower your chin to your chest and twist your head in a circular motion, bringing your ear to your shoulder and then returning to the beginning position. Repeat in the other direction. This technique relieves stress in the neck and improves neck mobility.

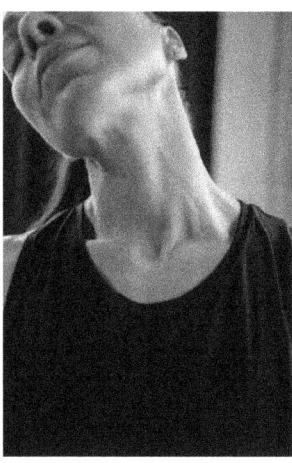

3. Shoulder Circles: Stand with your feet hip-width apart and your arms relaxed at your sides. Slowly roll your shoulders forward in a circular manner, then roll them backward. This practice relieves stress in the shoulders and improves shoulder mobility. See above chapter on "Arm Circles"

4. Spinal Twists: Sit on the floor, legs outstretched in front of you. Place your right hand on the floor behind you to provide support, and your left hand on your right knee. Gently rotate your body to the right and glance over your right shoulder. Hold for a few breaths, then repeat on the opposite side. This exercise relieves stress in the spine and improves spinal mobility.

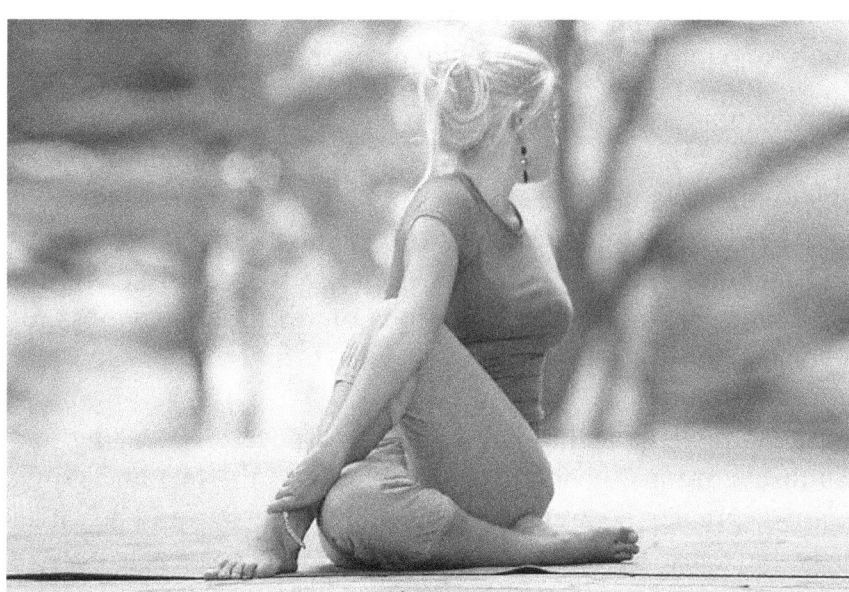

5. Breathing Exercises: Incorporating breathing exercises into your somatic practice is critical for increasing relaxation and awareness. Concentrate on deep, diaphragmatic breathing, allowing your belly to rise on inhalation and descend on exhalation. This may be done seated or laying down, focusing on the sensations of the breath as it flows in and out of your body. See above chapter also for illustration.

Building Awareness of Muscle Tension

Building awareness of muscle tension is a fundamental aspect of somatic practice. Muscle tension is a common part of our lives. It might result from regular activity, stress, emotional swings, or even bad posture. While some tension is normal, prolonged tightness can cause pain, discomfort, and restricted movement. Building awareness of this tension is the first step toward a calmer, balanced, and pain-free life.

Muscle tension is the condition of partial contraction in a muscle or set of muscles. It is a normal physiological reaction that can be triggered by stress, physical exercise, or prolonged use of a specific position. While some muscular tension is required for normal mobility and stability, persistent or excessive tension can cause discomfort, pain, and limited movement.

Why is Recognizing Muscle Tension Important?

- Pain and discomfort: Chronic tension can cause headaches, neck pain, backaches, and other musculoskeletal problems.
- Reduced mobility: Tight muscles limit your range of motion, which affects your daily activities and even exercise performance.
- Stress and anxiety: Muscle tension is frequently associated with stress and anxiety, generating a vicious cycle in which tension exacerbates stress and vice versa.
- Postural imbalances: Unbalanced muscular tension can cause poor posture, disrupting alignment and perhaps creating long-term issues.

Techniques for Building Awareness of Muscle Tension

Several techniques can help you tune into your body and identify areas of tension:

1. Body Scanning: Body scanning is a mindfulness method that entails gradually bringing awareness to various regions of the body. Individuals can mentally scan their bodies, beginning with the toes and progressing upward, noting areas of tension, pain, and relaxation. This technique promotes a more complete awareness of muscular tension throughout the body. Lie down comfortably and scan your body from head to toe, concentrating on any sensations of stiffness, heaviness, or pain. Pay attention to your breath and how it varies as you shift your focus to other regions.
2. Progressive Muscle Relaxation: This technique includes purposefully tensing and then relaxing specific muscle groups, generally beginning with the feet and going up. Individuals can gain a greater awareness of muscular tension and learn to release it spontaneously by consciously tensing and then relaxing each muscle group.
3. Breath Awareness: Paying attention to your breath might help you become more aware of muscle tightness. Individuals who breathe deeply and attentively can observe how the breath affects many regions of their bodies, particularly areas of stress. This can aid in identifying patterns of tension and relaxation related to breathing.

4. Mindful Movement: Gentle, mindful movements can also help you become more aware of muscular tightness. Individuals who move slowly and carefully can tune into the feelings in their muscles, detecting regions of tightness or limitation. This knowledge may then be utilized to modify movement patterns and reduce tension. Engage in gentle movements like yoga, tai chi, or qigong. Focus on the sensations in your muscles and joints as you move, noticing any areas of resistance or restriction.
5. Guided Imagery: This technique uses mental pictures or visions to induce relaxation and relieve stress. Individuals can increase their awareness of muscular tension and its potential for release by envisioning a tranquil, relaxing scenario or visualizing tension being released from specific muscles.
6. Self-massage: Gently massage areas that feel tight, using circular motions or light pressure. This can help release tension and improve circulation.
7. Journaling: Reflect on your daily activities and emotional state. Identify situations or emotions that trigger tension in your body, gaining insights into the psychological and physical connections.
8. Professional help: If you're struggling to manage muscle tension on your own, consider seeking help from a physiotherapist, massage therapist, or somatic practitioner. They can assess your body, provide personalized techniques, and address any underlying issues.

Tools to Relieve Tension

Once you've identified places of tension, you may use a variety of strategies to release:

Stretching: Gentle stretches in specific muscle areas can help lengthen and relax them, increasing flexibility and decreasing tension.

Breathing exercises: Deep, diaphragmatic breathing can activate your parasympathetic nervous system, promoting relaxation and releasing muscle tension.

Relaxation techniques: Practices such as progressive muscle relaxation or guided visualization can assist you in intentionally relaxing your muscles, reducing stress and tension.

Heat therapy: Using a heated pad on tense muscles helps increase blood flow and encourage relaxation.

Cold therapy: Icing acute tension points might decrease inflammation and give brief pain relief.

Chapter 5:

Intermediate Level Somatic Exercises

Intermediate-level somatic exercises expand on the fundamental concepts established in beginner practices, offering more complicated motions and sequences that test body awareness, coordination, and flexibility. These exercises are intended for people who have a fundamental knowledge of somatic concepts and are ready to graduate to more advanced activities. They seek to strengthen the mind-body connection, relieve deeper levels of stress, and modify movement patterns for better overall health. If you've already dipped your toes into the world of somatic movement and are craving deeper exploration, welcome to the realm of intermediate somatic exercises! Yes, you Welcome my reader

Here, you'll move beyond basic awareness and embark on a journey of refining your movement vocabulary, unlocking new possibilities, and fostering a deeper connection to your body's inner landscape. This chapter will delve into these aspects, providing a comprehensive understanding of how intermediate level somatic exercises can further enhance well-being and mindfulness.

Progressing to More Complex Movements

At the intermediate level, somatic exercises contain more complicated movement patterns that test coordination, balance, and flexibility. These motions may include integrating several aspects of somatic practice, such as breath synchronization, muscular relaxation, and conscious movement, into seamless sequences. By progressively introducing these intricacies, practitioners can improve their abilities and get a better knowledge of somatic concepts.

Deepening Body Awareness and Control

Intermediate-level somatic exercises focus on increasing body awareness and control. Practitioners learn to recognize subtle sensations and movement subtleties, resulting in a more refined awareness of their body's requirements and limits. This increased awareness allows practitioners to recognize and release deeper levels of stress, resulting in better general body function and movement quality.

Integrating Somatics into Daily Life

One of the fundamental aims of intermediate-level somatic practice is to incorporate somatic concepts into everyday living. Practitioners learn to incorporate the mindfulness and body awareness they develop during exercises into their daily routines. This integration enables a more holistic approach to well-being by incorporating somatic concepts into how people move, breathe, and interact with their surroundings.

What Makes Intermediate Somatic Exercises Different?

Intermediate practices expand on the basis of basic exercises, but with minor adjustments in emphasis and intensity:

- Greater complexity: Sequences may include more elaborate motions, such as rotations, spirals, and subtle weight distribution changes.
- Fascia exploration: You'll go deeper, focusing on the fascial system, which is an interwoven web of tissue that controls mobility and flexibility.
- Breath integration: As you move, your breath becomes more integrated, directing transitions and intensifying sensations.
- Emotional exploration: As your bodily awareness improves, more emotional layers may emerge, allowing for release and integration.

Ready to dive in? Here are some examples of intermediate somatic exercises to spark your practice:

1) Spinal Waves:

Lie on your back, knees bent, feet flat. Interlock your fingers behind your head.

Undulate your spine gently, starting at your tailbone and moving up through your vertebrae.

Imagine your spine as a gentle rippling wave on the ocean.

Breathe deeply and smoothly, linking your breath to the action.

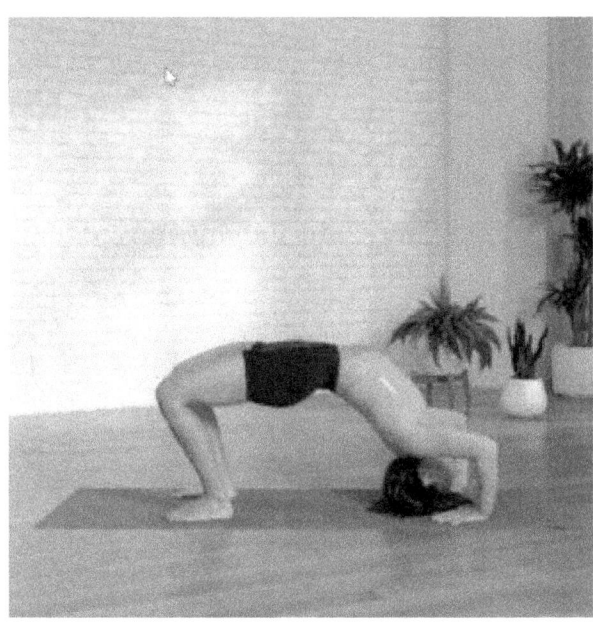

2. Facial release through rolling:

Sit on the floor, legs crossed. Put a tennis ball underneath your sitting bone.

Roll your body weight back and forth across the ball slowly and softly, focusing on the feelings in your hips and lower back.

Pay attention to regions of tightness or constriction and let your breath lead you as you relieve tension.

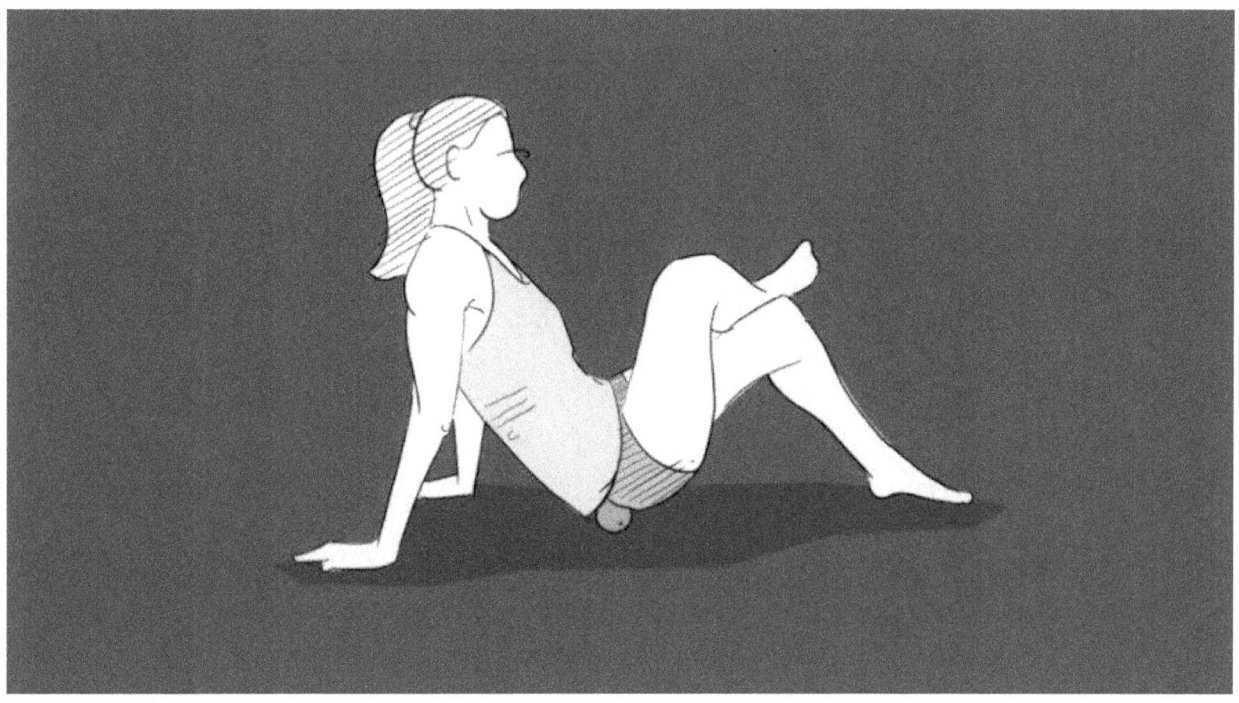

3. Breath-activated arm circles:

Stand hip-width apart, arms outstretched to the sides.

On an inhale, extend your arms upward, palms facing each other.

As you exhale, gradually pull your arms down and across your body, looping inward until they meet in front of your chest.

Repeat the action, matching your breath to the direction of your arms.

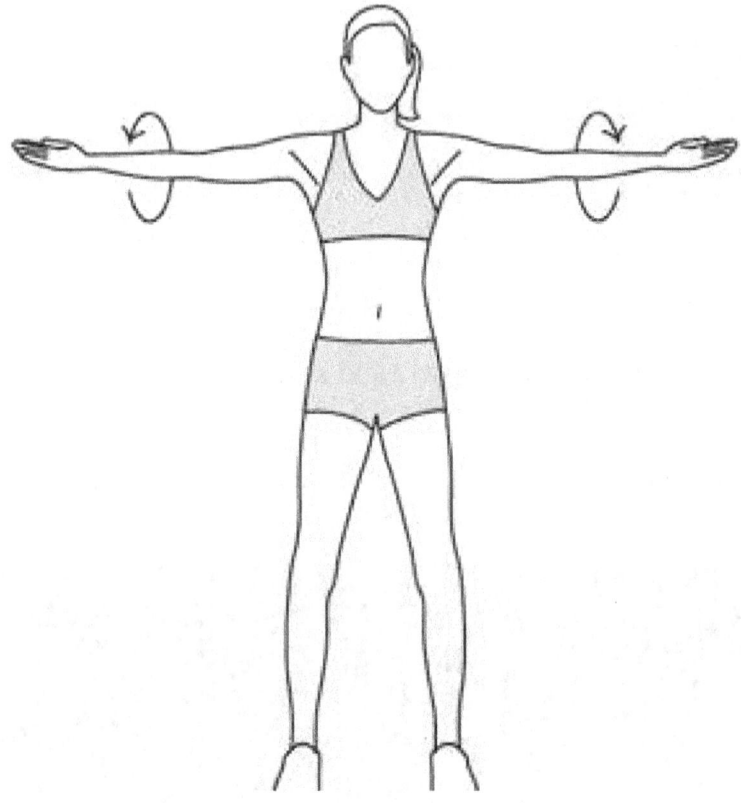

4. Emotional Release Through Movement:

Stand or sit comfortably, eyes closed. Take a few deep breaths and connect to your inner landscape.

Allow whatever feelings to emerge without judgment.

Express your feelings with delicate, spontaneous movements, allowing your body to guide you.

Take deep breaths and put your confidence in the movement and release process.

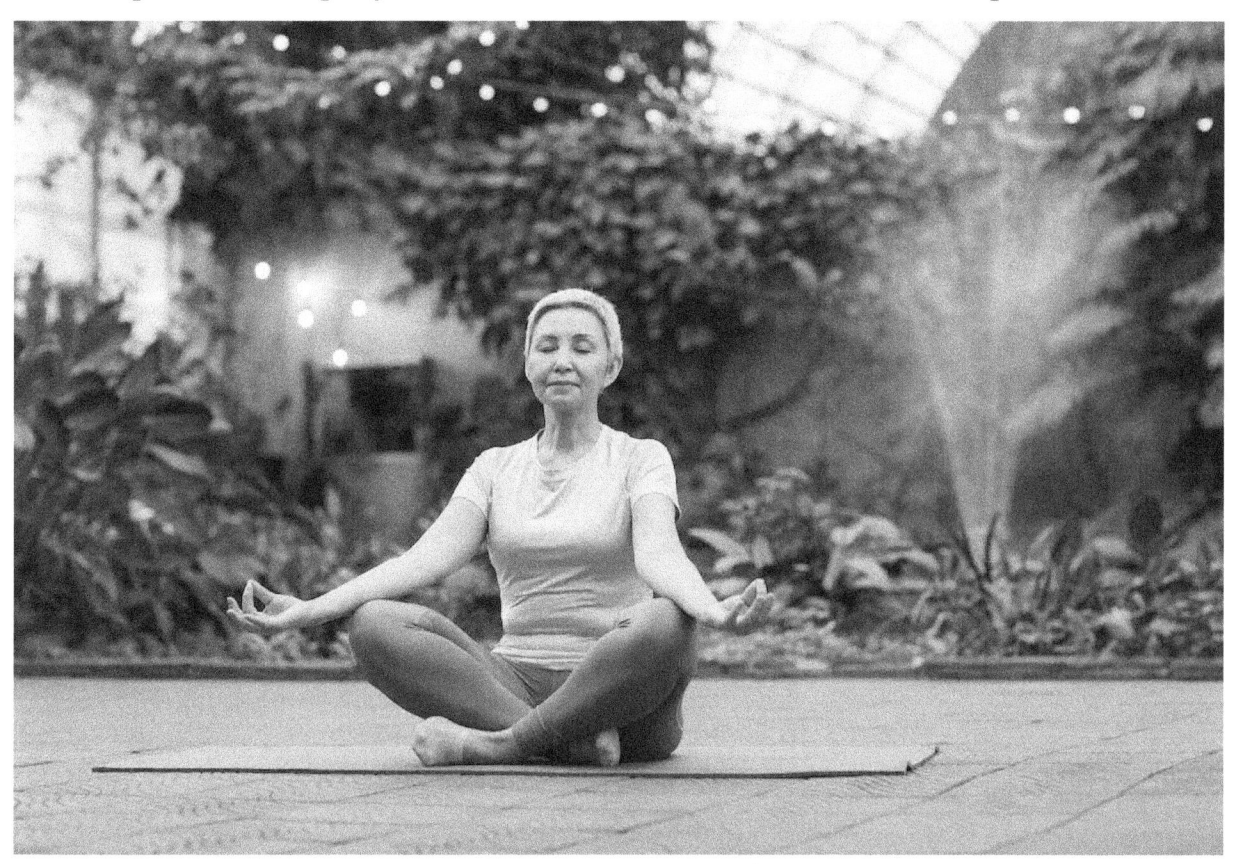

Remember:

Listen to your body and move with respect and care.

There is no right or wrong way to do these exercises. Focus on exploring and discovering what feels good for you.

Be patient and kind to yourself. Learning and integration take time.

Celebrate your progress and enjoy the journey of self-discovery!

Chapter 6: Advanced Level Somatic Exercises

In this chapter, we will look at the advanced level of somatic practice, in which practitioners refine movement patterns, challenge the body with complicated sequences, and incorporate somatic concepts into larger fitness routines. Advanced level somatic exercises are intended for people who have mastered the fundamental concepts of somatic practice and are ready to try more subtle and difficult motions. As you progress further into the realm of somatic movement, your practice evolves beyond fundamental awareness and into refinement, complexity, and self-discovery. Advanced somatic exercises take you beyond your comfort zone, encouraging you to explore complicated movement patterns, connect with your fascial system, and include breath and emotion into your movement language.

Challenging the Body with Advanced Sequences

Advanced somatic exercises include increasingly complicated and dynamic movement sequences that test the body's coordination, strength, and flexibility. These sequences may include somatic practice aspects with other movement modalities, such as yoga, Pilates, or dance, to provide a thorough and rigorous workout. Advanced sequences allow practitioners to develop their movement patterns and increase their body awareness.

Fine-Tuning Movement Patterns

At the advanced level, somatic exercises concentrate on fine-tuning movement patterns to improve efficiency, fluidity, and accuracy. Practitioners learn to improve their motor control and coordination, paying close attention to the nuances of movement and how each area of the body contributes to the total. This fine-tuning process can result in better overall movement quality and a stronger feeling of body awareness.

Incorporating Somatics into Fitness Routines

Advanced somatic exercises can be included into larger fitness regimens to improve overall performance and well-being. Practitioners can increase their movement efficiency, lower the chance of injury, and boost their overall fitness level by introducing somatic principles into activities like strength training, aerobic exercise, and sports-specific training. This integration enables a more holistic approach to fitness, with somatic practice being an essential component of a person's total training program.

What Sets Advanced Somatic Exercises Apart?

While expanding on the foundation of beginner and intermediate exercises, advanced practices have different characteristics:

- ❖ Increased Complexity: Movements become more intricate, incorporating combinations of rotations, spirals, subtle weight shifts, and variations in speed and intensity.
- ❖ Fascial Exploration: You'll learn more about your fascial system, the interwoven web of tissue that controls movement and flexibility, via movements that relieve tension and enhance mobility.
- ❖ Breath Integration: Breathing becomes an essential component of your movements, directing transitions, heightening sensations, and fostering a stronger mind-body connection.
- ❖ Emotional Exploration: As your physical awareness improves, more emotional layers may emerge, providing possibilities for release and integration via mindful movement.

Are you ready to ascend? Example of Advanced Somatic Exercises:

1. Dynamic Transition:

Move effortlessly between different postures or exercises, concentrating on the transitions as much as the poses. This promotes fluidity and awareness of movement changes.

2. Facial Release with Self-Massage:

Tennis balls, foam rollers, and other instruments can be used to alleviate tension in your body's numerous fascial lines. Pay attention to regions of tension and take deep breaths as you release.

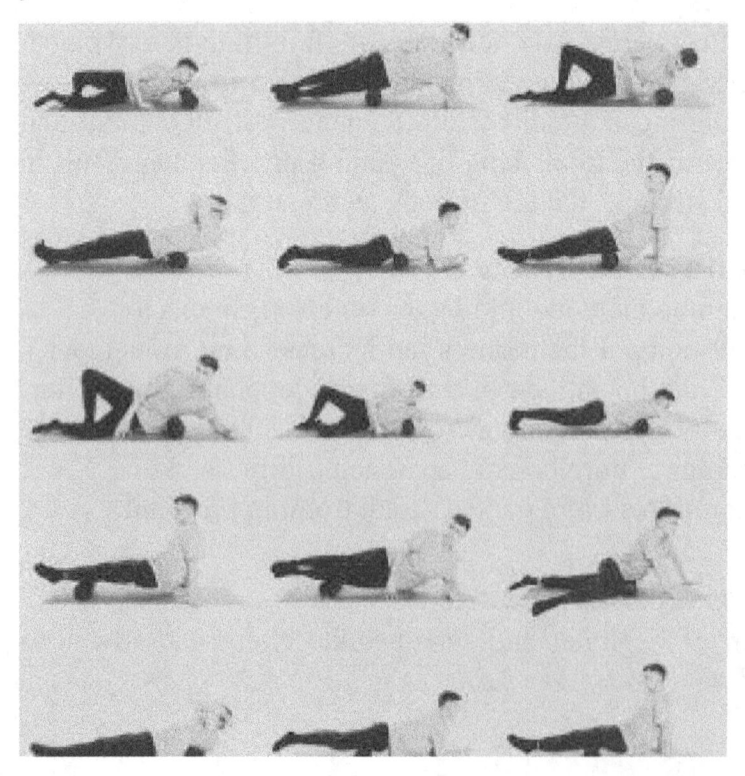

3. Breathwork and Movement:

Combine particular breathing methods, such as Kapalbhati or Bhastrika, with dynamic movements to investigate the relationship between breath and movement. Examine how breathing affects your energy levels and movement quality.

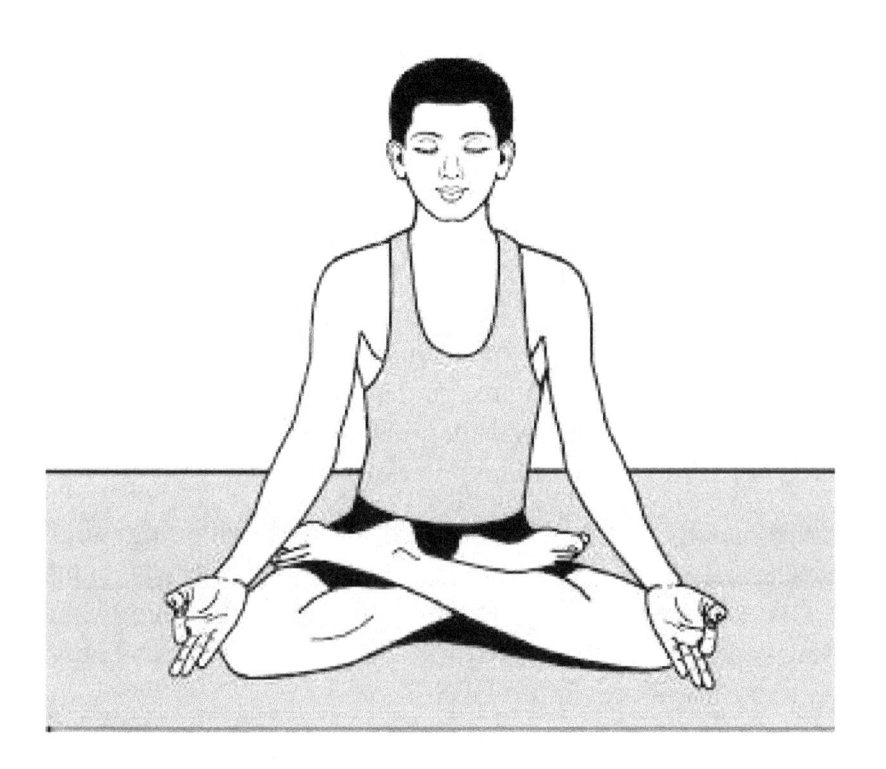

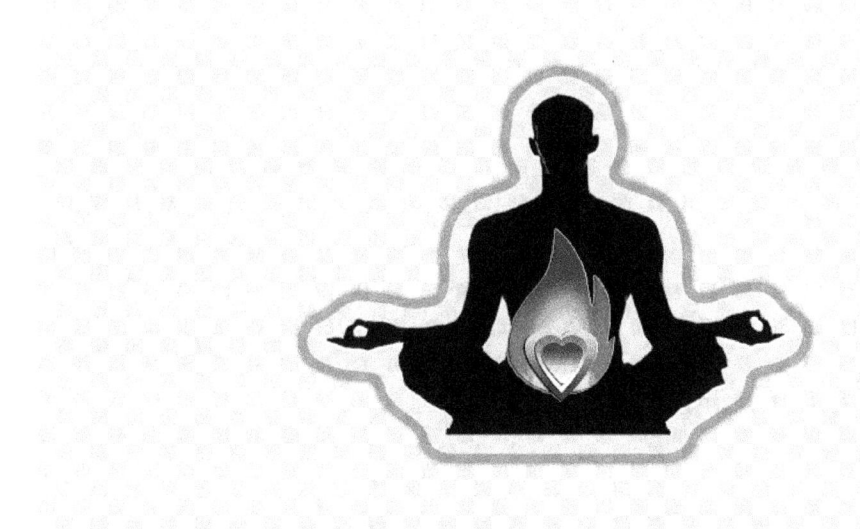

43 | Somatic Exercises for Beginners

4. Partnered Somatic Exploration: Work with a trusted partner to gently coach each other through dance sequences while offering feedback and encouragement. This encourages greater self-awareness and connection.

5. Somatic Meditation in Motion: Combine contemplative awareness and mild, attentive movements. Focus on your body's feelings without judgment, allowing movement to emerge organically.

Expanding your horizons:

As you master these advanced exercises, try branching out into specific areas of somatic practice:

Laban Movement Analysis: Laban movement analysis (LMA), also known as Laban/Bartenieff movement analysis, is a method and vocabulary used to describe, visualize, analyze, and document human movement. It is based on Rudolf Laban's original work, which was refined and expanded by Lisa Ullmann, Irmgard Bartenieff, Warren Lamb, and others. LMA draws from a variety of disciplines, including anatomy, kinesiology, and psychology. Dancers, actors, musicians, and athletes utilize it, as do health professionals including physical and occupational therapists and psychotherapists, as well as in anthropology, business consulting, and leadership development.

Examines movement characteristics such as flow, space, and time, broadening your movement vocabulary. Laban classified motions as Eukinetics, or Efforts, and Choreutics, or Space Harmony. His work was continued on, notably by Bartenieff and Ullmann, and classified into four categories: body, effort, shape, and space. These categories are commonly referred to by the abbreviation BESS.

Body

This relates to what the physical form is doing—such as movement independence or interconnectivity—as well as how movement is transferred from one portion of the body to another.

Effort

Laban identified eight basic ways in which movement produces experience or feeling. These Efforts are divided into four motion factors: space, time, weight, and flow, which represent how your body moves through the world. He also created two aspects for each Effort to explain its characteristics: space (or direction) is either direct or indirect; time (or speed) is either fast or sustained; weight is either heavy or light; and flow is either constrained or free. The eight Effort acting techniques are:

- Dab: direct, rapid, light, bound.
- Float: indirect, continuous, light and free
- Press: direct, sustained, heavy, and bound
- Wring: indirect, persistent, heavy, and bound.

- Glide: straight, steady, light and free
- Punch: straight, rapid, heavy, bound.
- Slash: indirect, rapid, heavy, free.
- Flick: indirect, rapid, light, free.

Shape

This explains how and why your body changes shape. Subcategories include:

Shape forms are your body's fixed shapes.

Modes of form change: how your body interacts with its surroundings. The modes include "shape flow," or your body's connection to itself; "directional," or your body's orientation within its surroundings; and "carving," or your body's interaction with the size of the environment.

form flow support refers to how your core or torso changes form to support the rest of your body.

Space

This describes how your body fills the area around it, particularly harmoniously. Aspects include:

Kinesphere: the physical space surrounding your body and how you react to it.

Spatial intention: how you, the mover, employ distinct directions.

Body Mind Centering: Body-Mind Centering (BMC) is a continuous, experiential journey into the living and changing realm of the body. The explorer is our mind, which includes our ideas, feelings, energy, soul, and spirit. Throughout this trip, we get an awareness of how the mind expresses itself via the body in movement. Combines movement with anatomical structures and images to enhance your awareness of your body.

Chapter 7: 30-Day Somatic Exercise Routine

Day 1: **Diaphragmatic Breathing** **TIME: 30 MINUTES**

This exercise helps to activate your body's relaxation response. It involves deep breathing into the diaphragm rather than shallow breathing from your chest.

Steps:
1. Lie or sit comfortably.
2. Place one hand on your stomach, the other on your chest.
3. Take a slow, deep breath in through your nose, feeling your tummy rise as you fill your lungs with air. The hand on your chest should be as motionless as possible.
4. Exhale gently via your mouth or nose, allowing your tummy to descend.
5. Repeat for a few minutes.

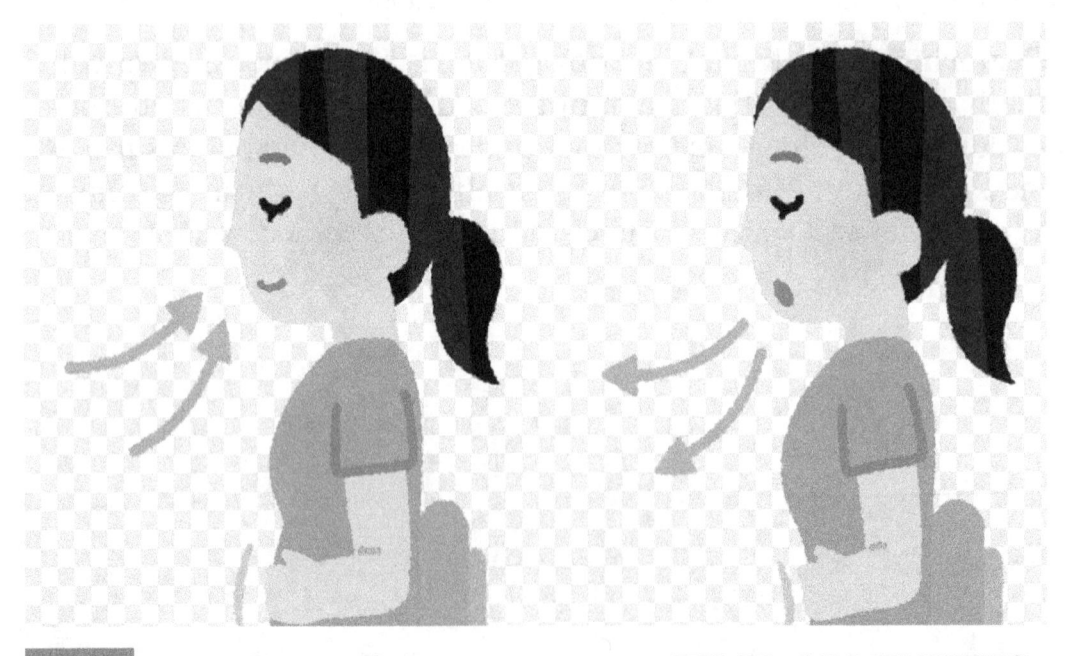

Illustration:

Day 2: **Grounding** **TIME: 25 MINUTES**

Grounding techniques can help you feel more connected to your physical presence in the world.

Steps:

1. Stand up straight and feel your feet firmly planted on the earth. Taking your shoes off for this workout may make you feel more relaxed.
2. Take a few deep breaths, concentrating on the sensation of your feet connecting to the ground.
3. Imagine roots emerging from your feet, attaching you to the ground, and feeling linked to the soil.
4. Start moving your weight from left to right, swaying like a tree.
5. Shift your weight from front to rear.
6. As you transfer your weight, pay attention to your center of gravity, which is positioned in the upper pelvis and below the navel.
7. Place your hands on top of your lower tummy and feel the center.
8. Continue to sway from side to side and front to back, keeping your hands on top of your lower abdomen.

Illustration:

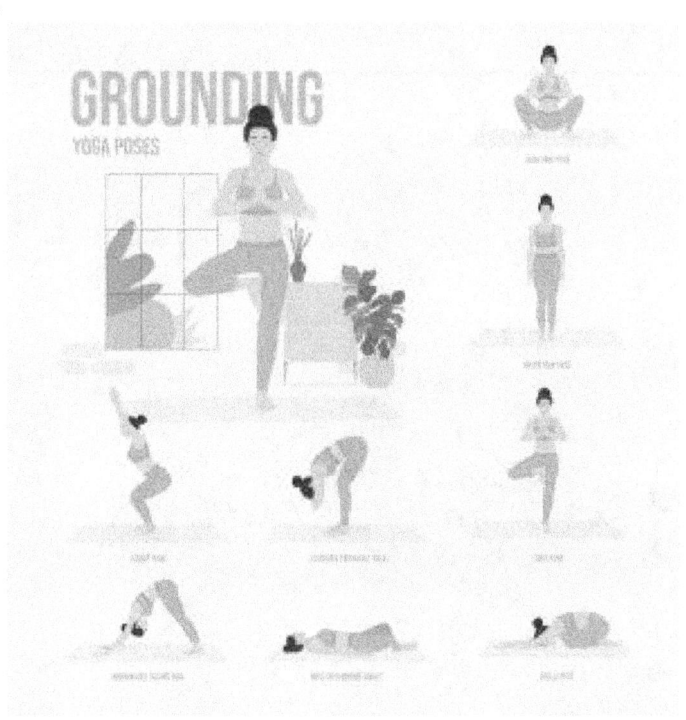

Day 3:   Body Scanning   TIME: 15 MINUTES

This technique promotes increased bodily awareness and can help identify areas of tension or discomfort.

Steps:

1. Lie or sit comfortably.
2. Mentally examine your body from toes to head, noting any points of tension or discomfort.
3. Spend a few seconds focusing on each location, and if you notice any tightness, breathe deeply and exhale, allowing the area to relax.
4. When you feel the body part relax, go to the next one.
5. Continue the technique until you reach your head.

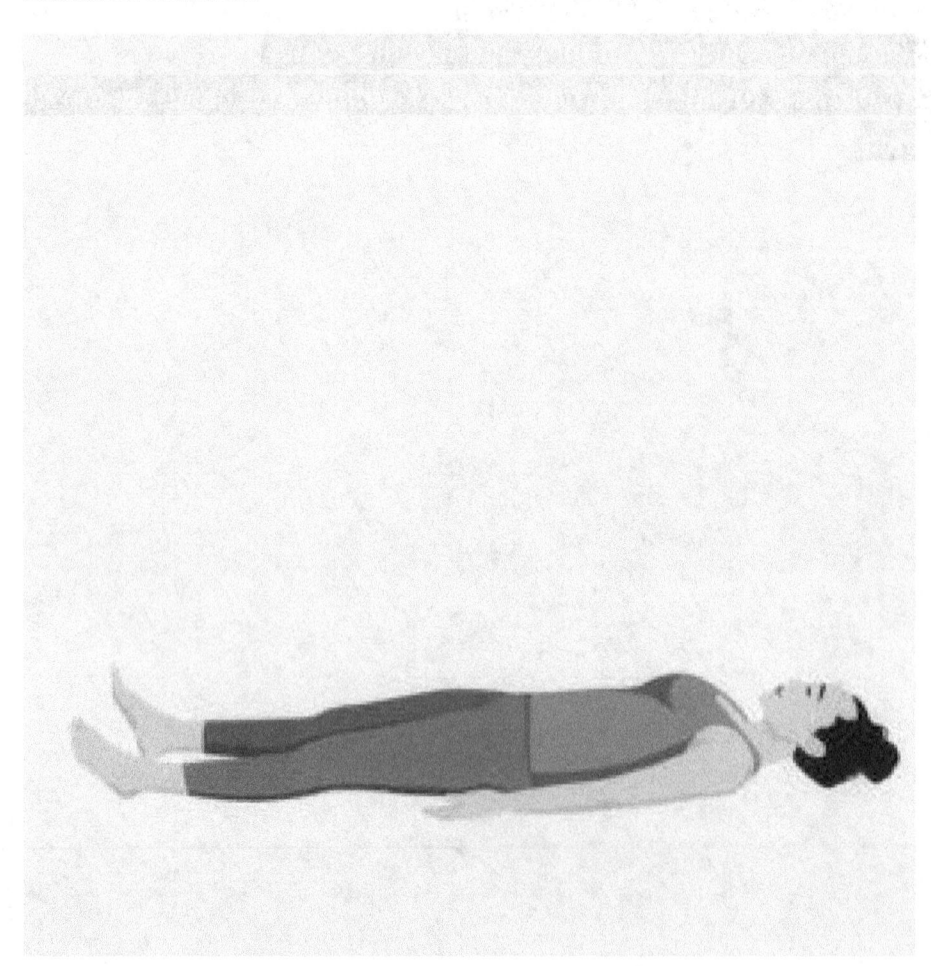

Illustration:

Day 4: Fascial Release with Rolling   TIME: 15 MINUTES

It can help relieve muscle tightness, soreness, and inflammation, and increase your joint range of motion.

Steps:

1. Sit on the floor, legs crossed, with a tennis ball beneath your sitting bone.
2. Gently move your body weight back and forth, focusing on the feelings in your hips and lower back.
3. Take deep breaths and let go of whatever stress you're feeling.
4. Switch sides and repeat.
5. Roll both forearms on a tennis ball from wrist to elbow, concentrating on tight spots.

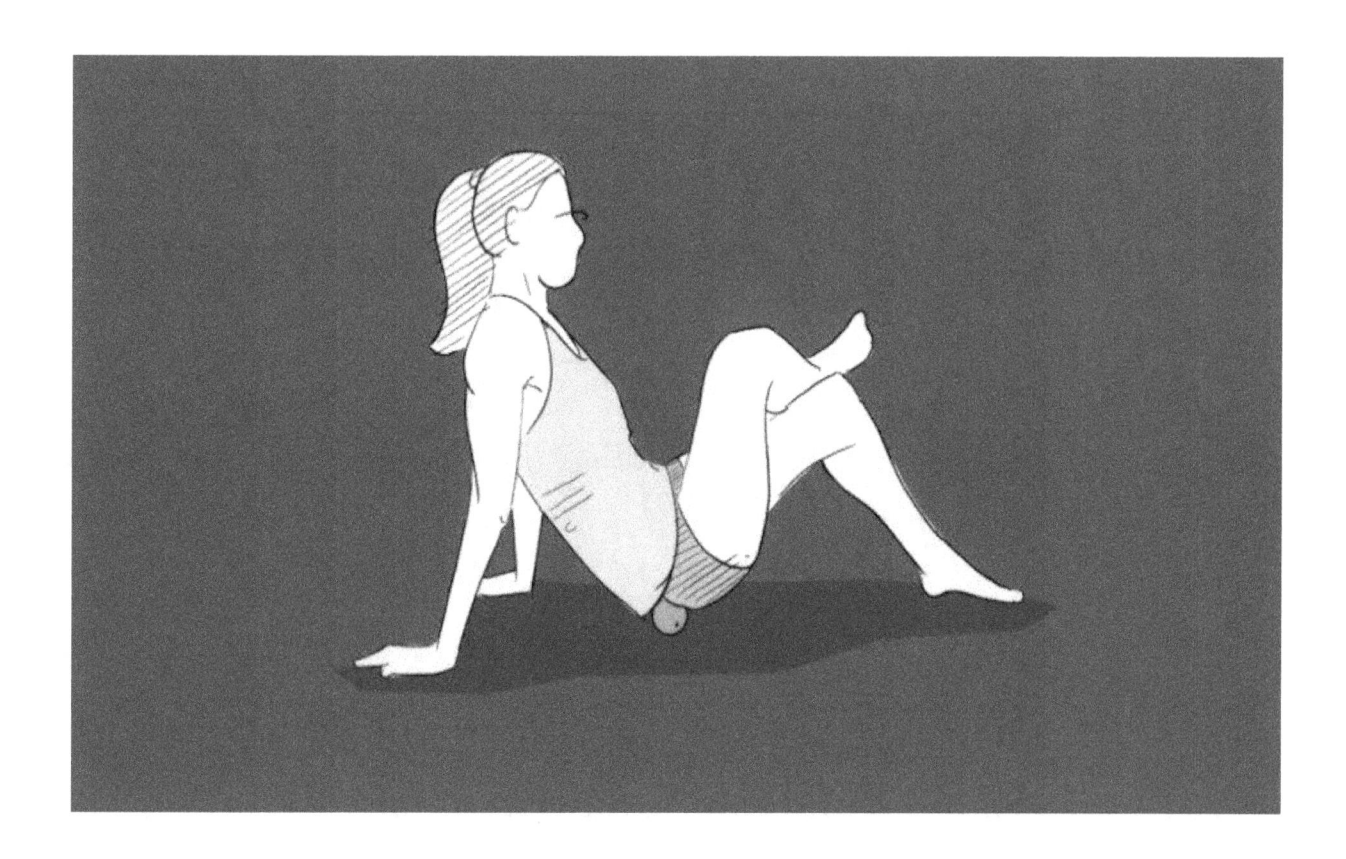

Illustration:

Day 5: Breathwork & Arm Circles — TIME: 15 MINUTES

What exactly happens when you circle your arms?

Arm circles can help tone the muscles in your shoulder and arm, namely the biceps and triceps. They also target your upper back muscles.

Steps:

1. Stand hip-width apart, arms outstretched to the sides.
2. Inhale deeply and raise your arms upwards, palms facing each other.
3. Exhale gently, bringing your arms down and across your body, then looping inwards till they meet in front of your chest.
4. Repeat the action, matching your breath to the direction of your arms. Close your eyes and concentrate on the feelings in your body while breathing

Illustration:

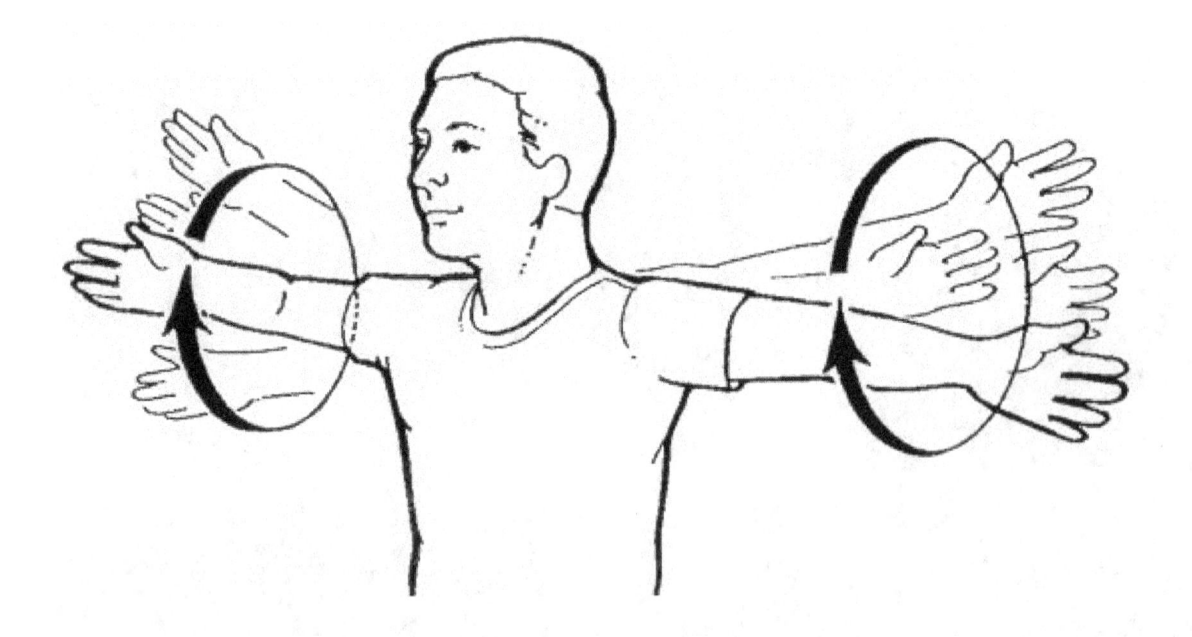

PRACTICE TO PERFECTION! KEEP GOING READER

Day 6: Pelvic Tilts & Spinal Waves TIME: 15 MINUTES

Pelvic tilting exercises are commonly used to improve the alignment of the lumbar spine of individuals with chronic lower back pain (LBP).

Steps:

1. Lie on your back, legs bent, feet flat on the floor.
2. Press your lower back into the mat and tilt your pelvis up to engage your core.
3. Hold for a few seconds, then gently release. Repeat 5-10 times.
4. Lie on your back, legs bent, feet flat on the floor.
5. Undulate your spine gently, starting at your tailbone and moving up through your vertebrae.
6. Imagine your spine as a gentle rippling wave on the ocean.

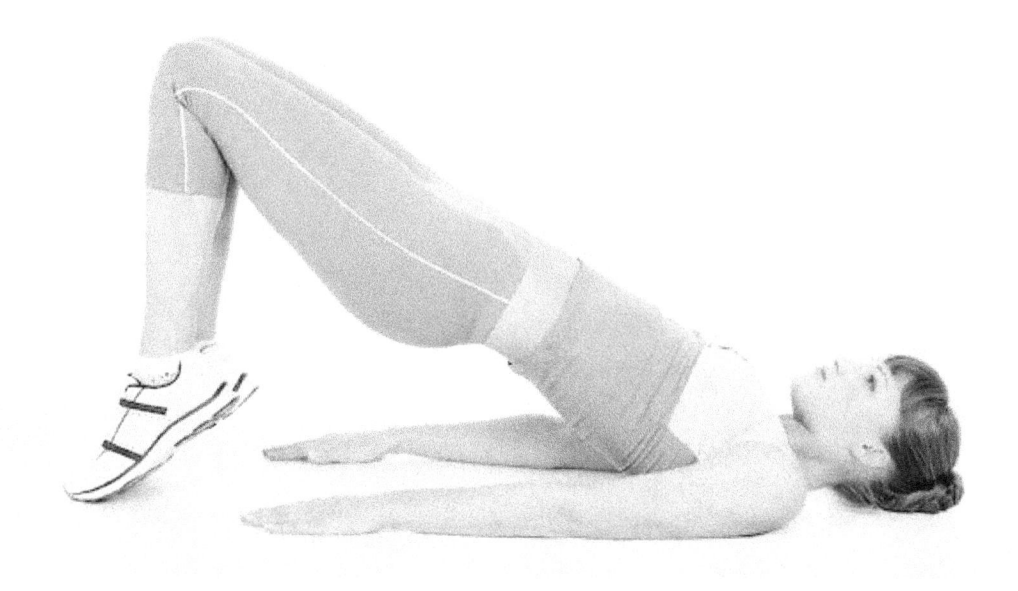

Illustration:

Day 7: **Rest & Reflection (Free Day)**   **TIME: HOURS**

Engage in mindful movement throughout the day, such as stretching, walking, dancing, or simply listening to your body. Consider your adventure thus far. Note any insights or observations.

Wrap it Up at the end of each week!

Day 8: SENSORY AWARENESS   TIME: 30 MINUTES

This practice promotes greater awareness of your sensory experiences.

Steps:

1. Choose a quiet area to sit or lie down.
2. Close your eyes and take several deep breaths.
3. Tune in to each of your senses, focusing for a few seconds on what you can hear, smell, feel, taste, and see (with your eyes closed).

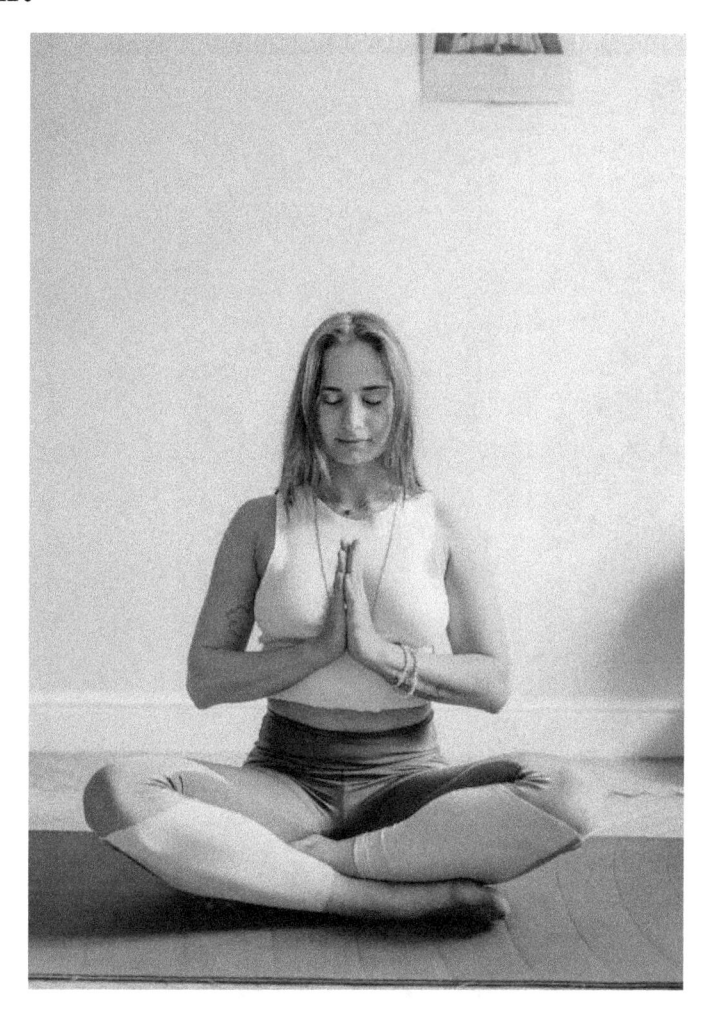

Illustration:

Day 9: The Voo Breath   TIME: 15 MINUTES

This voice practice can activate your vagus nerve, resulting in a sensation of peace and relaxation.

Steps:

1. Find a comfortable location and settle into a comfortable position, whether sitting on a chair or on the floor.
2. Focus your attention on your physiological feelings and the current moment. Take note of how you breathe in and out.
3. Draw a big breath in.
4. As you exhale, create a "voo" sound, holding the vowel for as long as possible. This sound will vibrate throughout your abdomen and chest.
5. Repeat a few times.

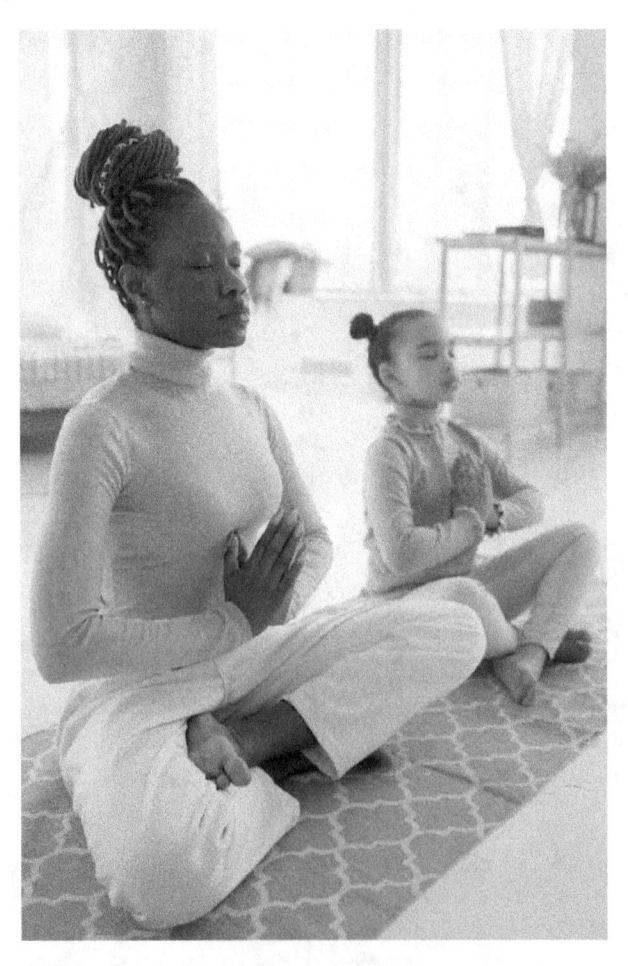

Illustration:

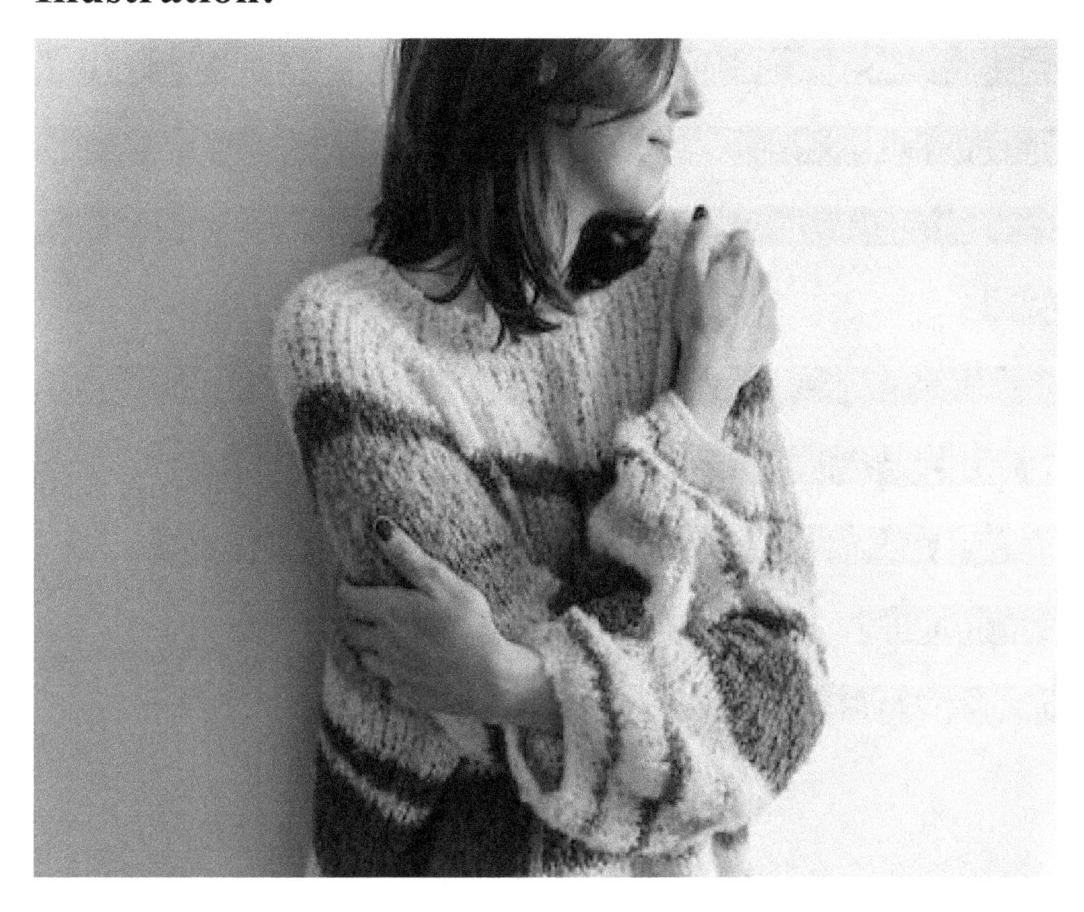

Day 10: Self-Hug   TIME: 15 MINUTES

This calming technique can assist to alleviate discomfort.

Steps:

1. Cross your right arm across your chest to feel your heartbeat, and rest your left hand on your right shoulder.
2. Apply mild pressure and rock from side to side.
3. Take deep, soothing breaths while holding this self-hug.

Illustration:

Day 11: Eagle Poses TIME: 15 MINUTES

Facilitates deep breathing. Wrapping your arms in front of you opens up the back of your lungs, allowing you to breathe more deeply.

Steps:

1. Transfer your weight to your left foot.
2. Lift your right foot off the floor.
3. Cross your right thigh across your left as far up the thigh as possible.
4. Hook your right foot around your left calf.
5. Bring both arms out in front of you, parallel to the ground.
6. Bend your arms and cross the left arm across the right, connecting the elbows. With your arms hooked, bring your forearms together and wrap your right hand around your left, crossing at the wrists. (If one leg is on top, the other arm should be on top.)
7. Lift your elbows to the height of your shoulders, but maintain your shoulders down and away from your ears.
8. Maintain a perpendicular spine to the floor, with the top of the head rising.
9. Hold for 5-10 breaths.
10. Repeat on the opposite side.

Illustration: Eagle Pose

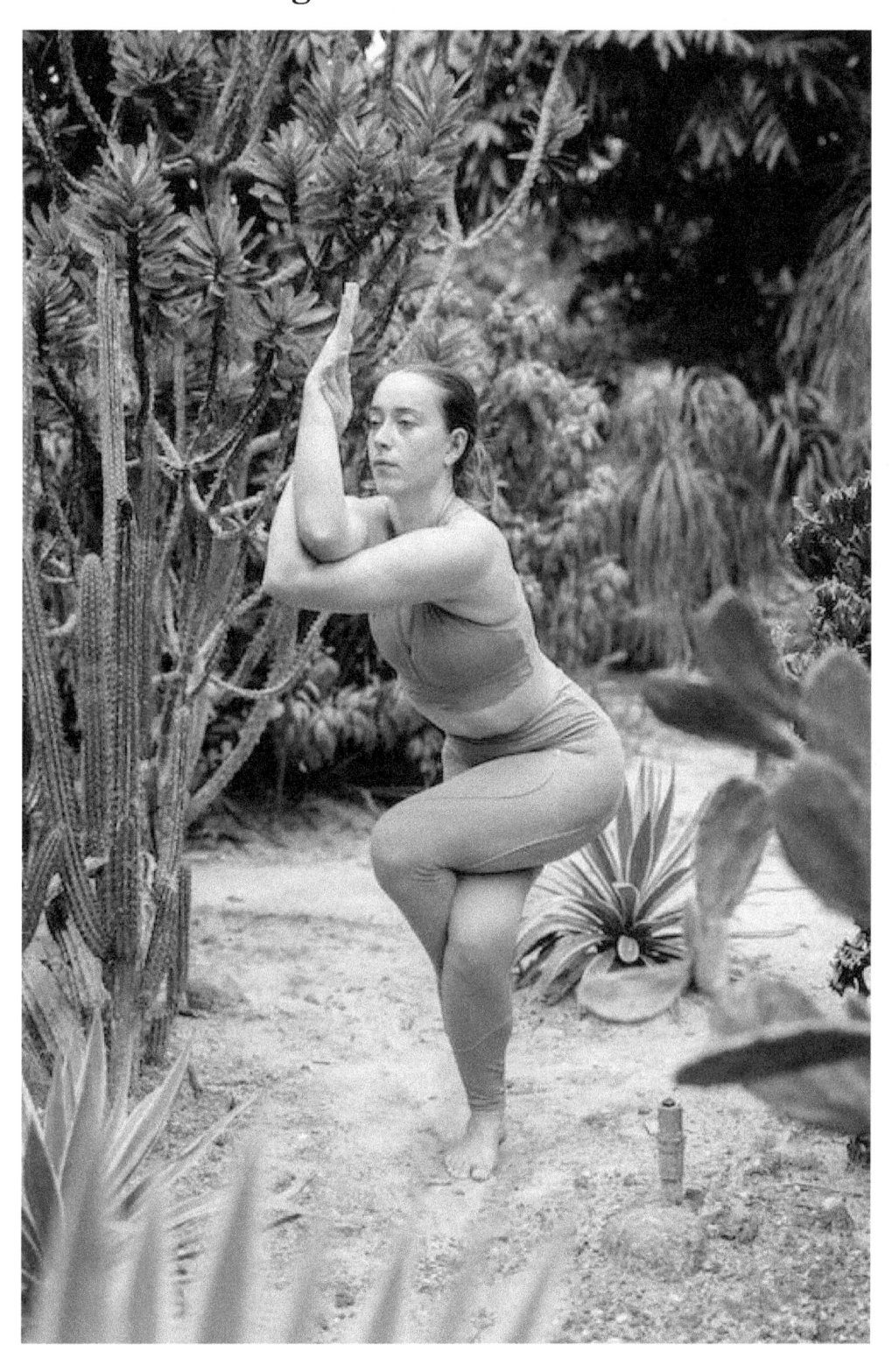

Day 12: Superman   TIME: 20 MINUTES

Among other benefits, the Superman stance promotes strong posture. As Healthline says, the more you can strengthen your core and back muscles, the more support your spine will receive!

Steps:

1. Lie on the floor in a prone (facedown) posture, legs straight, arms outstretched in front of you.

2. Keeping your head in a neutral posture (avoid looking up), steadily raise your arms and legs about 6 inches (15.3 cm) off the floor, or until you feel your lower back muscles tense. Engage your glutes, core, and the muscles between your shoulder blades at the same time.

3. Lift your belly button slightly off the floor to compress your abs. Imagine yourself as Superman, flying through the air.

4. Hold this posture for 2–3 seconds. Make careful to breathe the entire time.

5. Lower your arms, legs, and belly to the floor. Repeat the exercise for 2-3 sets of 8-12 repetitions.

Illustrations: Superman

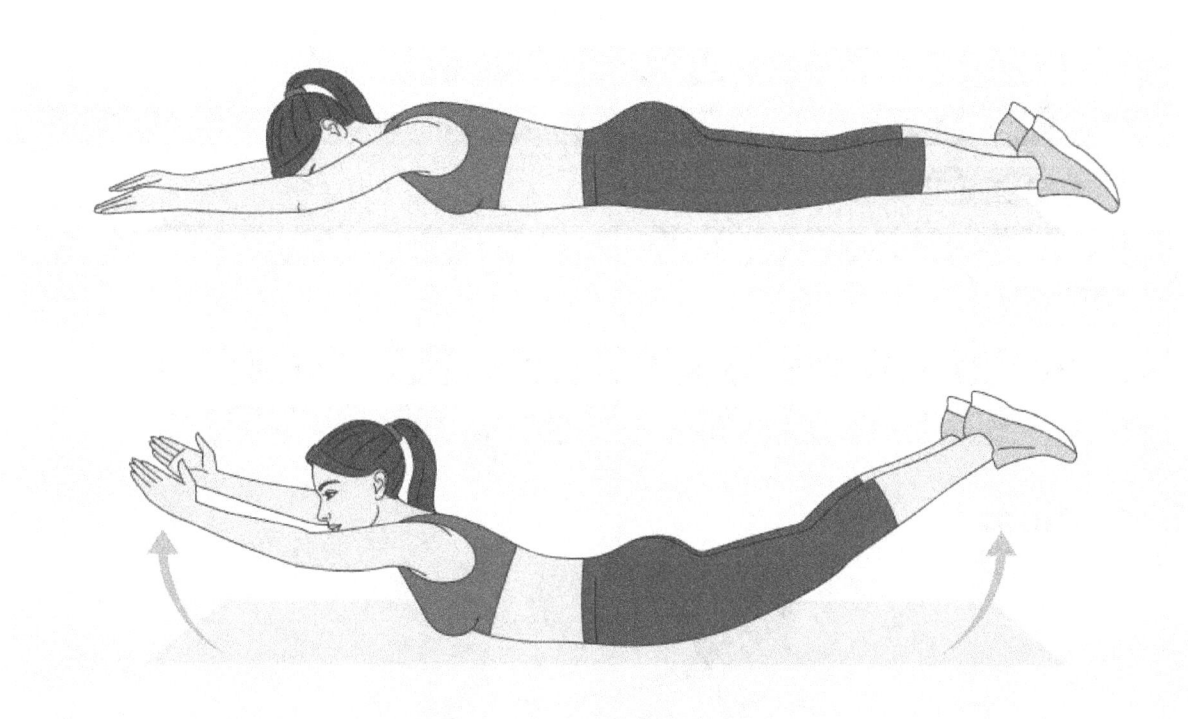

PRACTICE TO PERFECTION! KEEP GOING READER

Day 13: Knee Hold   TIME: 15 MINUTES

This exercise helps to prevent your knee from getting chronically twisted.

Steps:

1. Use a solid workout platform that is no higher than 6 inches.
2. Place one foot on the platform and step up, bringing the second foot up near to it but not upon it.
3. Hold this stance for up to 5 seconds, focusing your weight on the foot on the platform.
4. Slowly return the "floating" foot to the floor, followed by the other foot.
5. Repeat 5-10 times before switching sides and doing another 5-10 times.

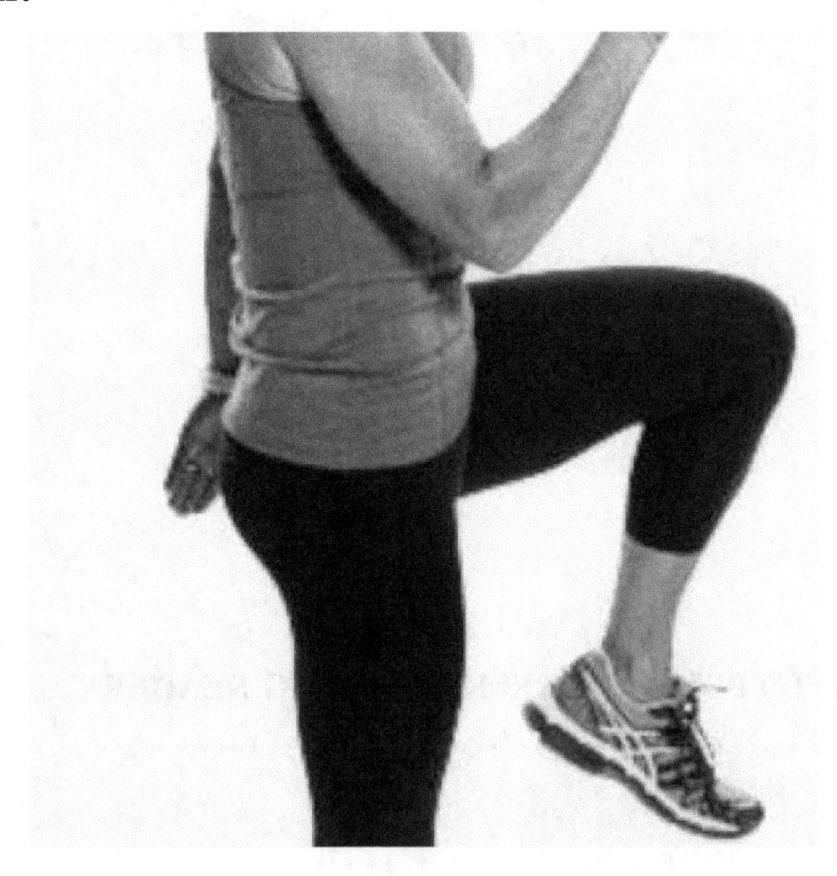

Illustration:

Day 14: **Rest & Reflection (Free Day)** **TIME: HOURS**

Engage in mindful movement throughout the day, such as stretching, walking, dancing, or simply listening to your body. Consider your adventure thus far. Note any insights or observations.

Wrap it Up at the end of each week!

Day 15: Jumping Jacks   TIME: 25 MINUTES

Jumping jacks raise your heart rate and burn calories, which helps to reduce overall body fat, including belly fat.

Steps:

1. Stand erect with your feet together and your hands by your sides.

2. Begin the exercise by lifting your hands over your head and springing up just enough to split your feet twice shoulder width apart.

3. Reverse the movement back to the starting position without halting. Repeat as many times as needed, as soon as possible.

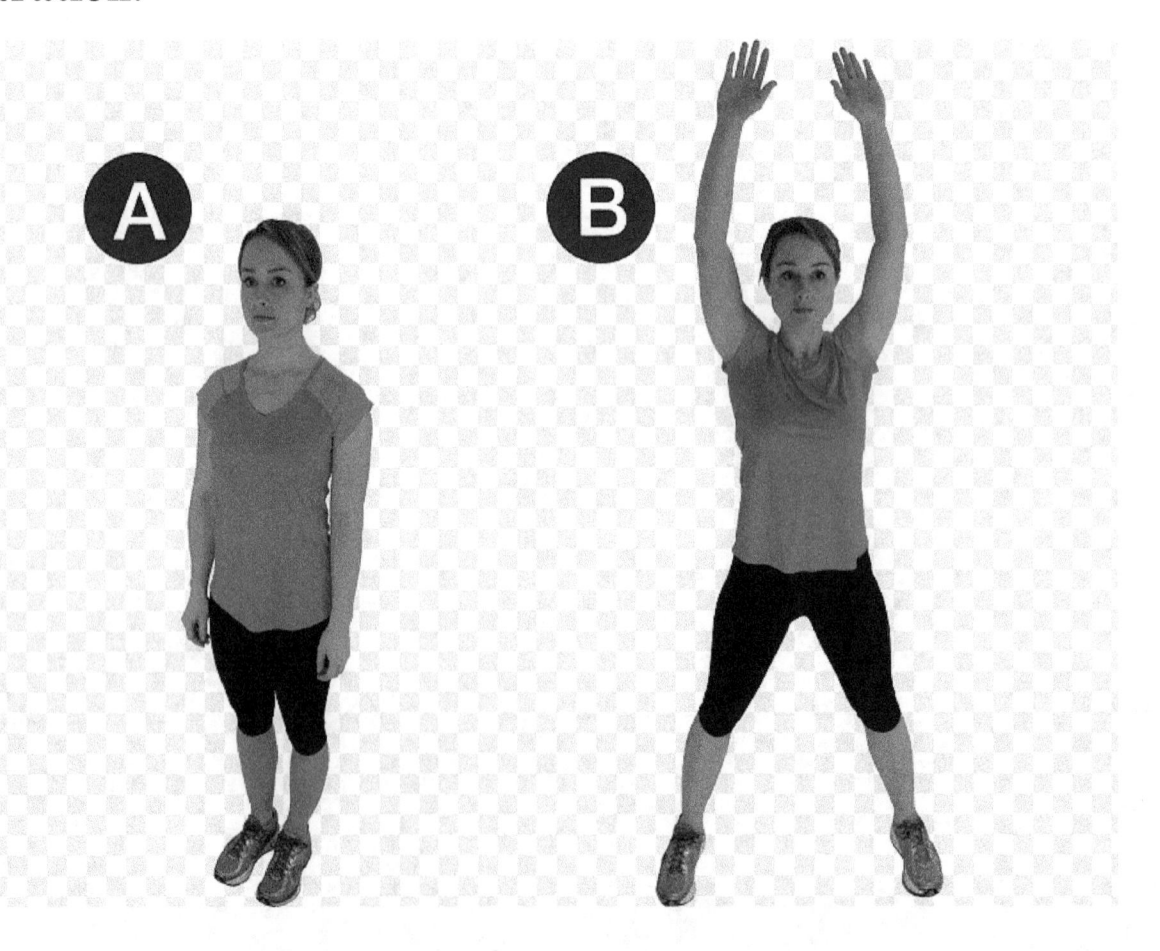

Illustration:

Day 16: Reach Back   TIME: 25 MINUTES

This exercise focuses on indirectly improving hand behind back motion by moving and stretching other areas, including the opposite pec muscles. Try it out and see how your hand behind the back motion is before and after!

Steps:

1. Begin by going down on all fours (hands and knees). Keep your back straight, bend one elbow, and rest your hand on the back of your head.
2. Start the exercise by attempting to contact your elbow to the opposing knee. After you've gone as far down as you can, spin up such that your elbow points to the ceiling.
3. Go up to the count of two and then down to the count of two. Perform three sets of eight to ten repetitions on each side. As you gain strength, attempt to increase the number of repetitions as the weeks pass.

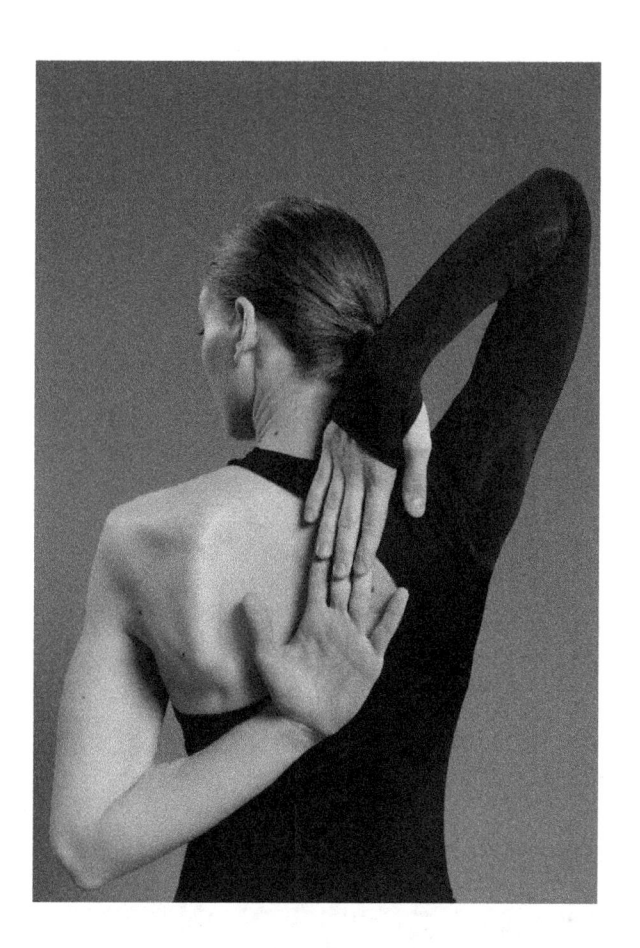

Illustration:

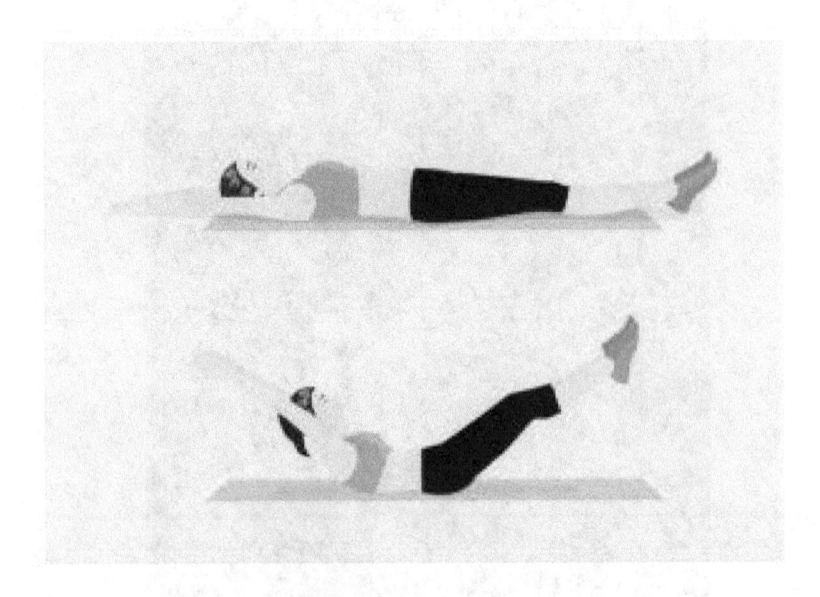

Day 17: Body Rocking — TIME: 30 MINUTES

It may be done as a warm-up exercise to help engage your core, throughout a workout as a strengthening component, or as a finisher at the end of a session.

Steps:

1. Lie on your back. Reach toward the ceiling with both arms, lifting your shoulder blades off the floor. Your arms should be in line with your ears, fully stretched straight out.
2. Push your lower back to the floor and elevate your legs 3 to 6 inches off the ground while maintaining your toes pointed. Create tension by squeezing your legs, arms, and abs together.
3. Begin to rock back and forth, maintaining tension so as not to break the arch formed by your legs and arms. Keep your abs engaged throughout.
4. Repeat as many times as possible with proper form.

Illustration:

Day 18: Side Reach   TIME: 30 MINUTES

Regular side stretches can help you gain flexibility and range of motion. This exercise elongates and strengthens certain muscle groups, allowing for increased ease of movement in regular tasks.

Steps:

1. Stand tall with your feet hip-width apart or slightly further apart (a broader stance makes it easier to balance). Place your left hand at your side, palm contacting your thigh.

2. Raise your right hand high over your head and completely stretch your elbow and shoulder. Point your fingers towards the sky.

3. Keep your right arm up and lean to the left. Continue to lean and lower your left hand until you feel a tug on the right side of your body.

4. Allow your neck to lower and sink into the stretch.

5. Stay here for five to ten seconds before returning to your starting point.

6. Repeat on the opposite side.

7. Continue alternating for 10 to 20 repetitions. Complete two to three sets for a stretch exercise that provides long-lasting relief from tension.

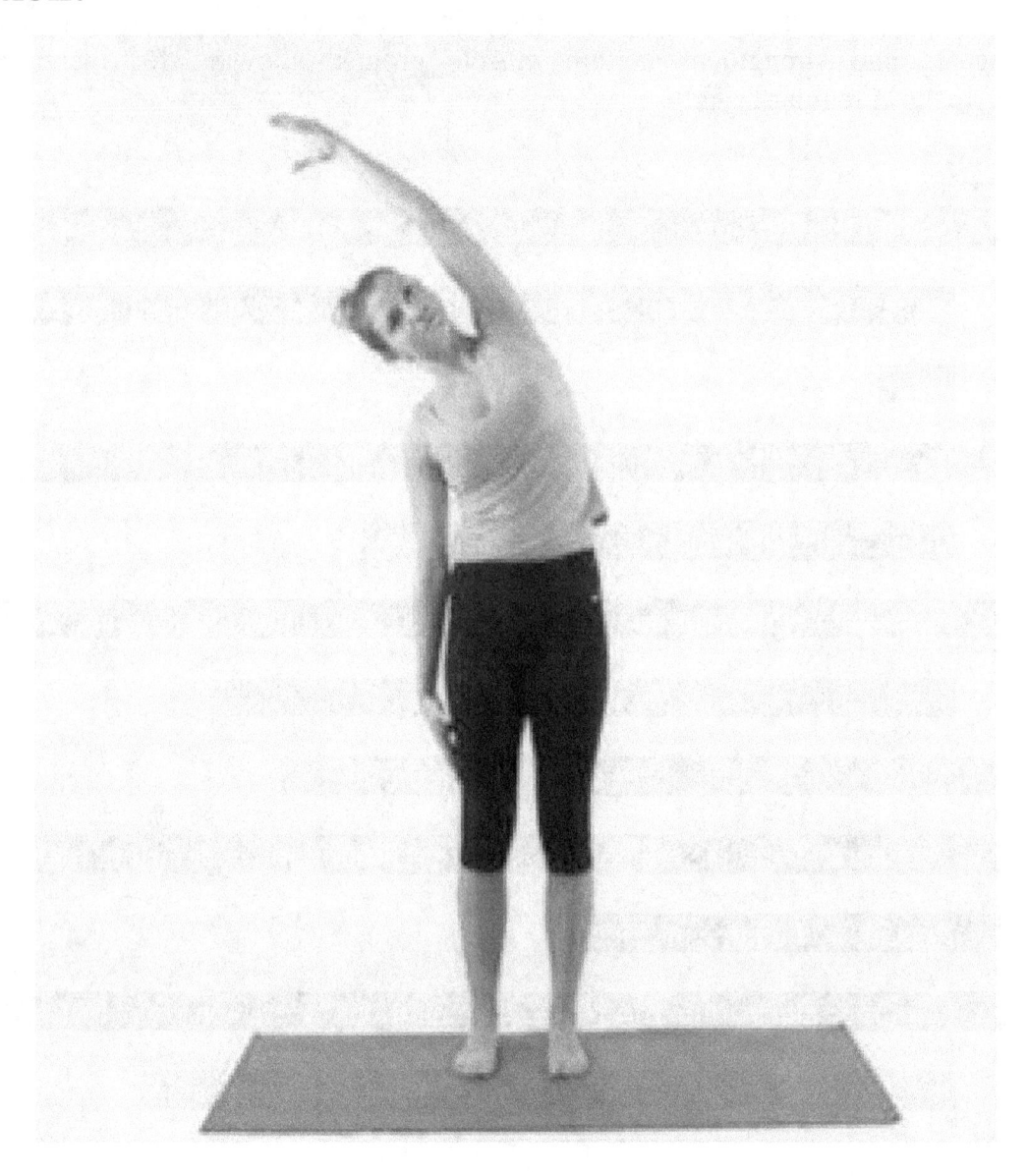

Illustration:

PRACTICE TO PERFECTION! KEEP GOING READER

Day 19: Hip Circles   TIME: 30 MINUTES

Hip circles entail moving your hips in a circular way. It strengthens your hips and core muscles. It helps to improve flexibility and balance. Start with small circles and gradually increase the size to challenge yourself.

Steps:

1. Stand on one leg, relying on a countertop or wall for support.
2. Swing your other leg in little circles out to the side.
3. Perform 20 circles, then swap legs.
4. As you gain flexibility, gradually increase the size of your circles.

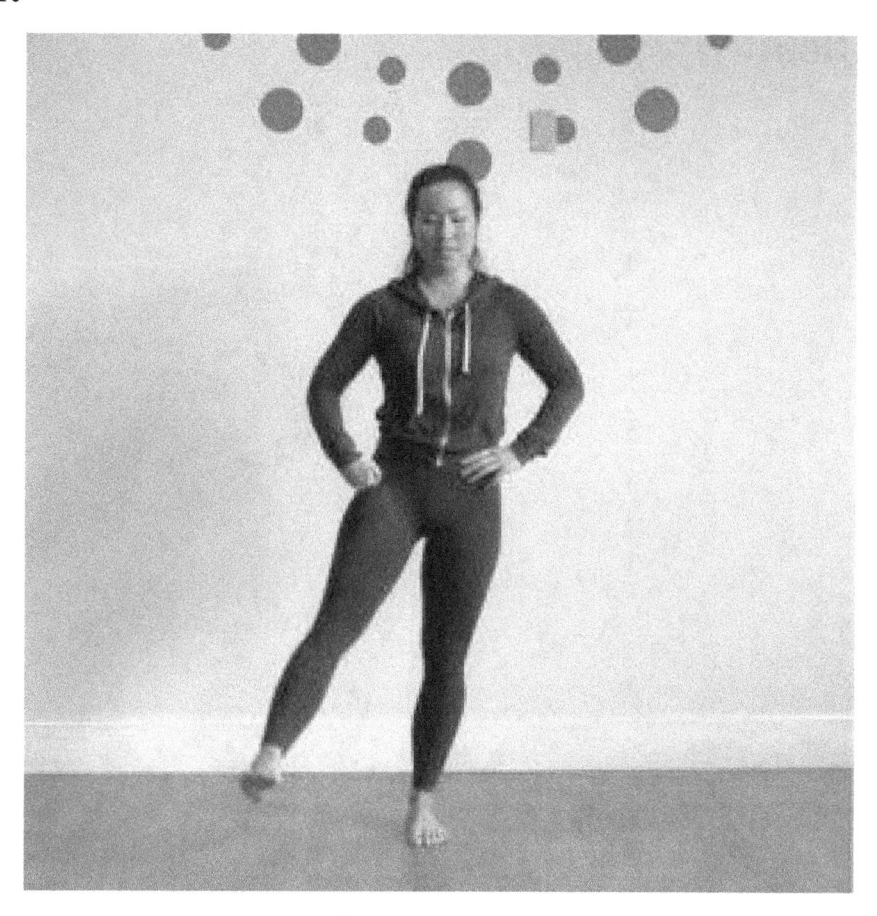

Illustration:

Day 20: Spinal Rotations TIME: 30 MINUTES

A mild twist of the spine mobilizes the back while simultaneously stretching the shoulders and heart region. In this approach, tensions can be relieved. The twist massages the digestive organs (liver and kidney), stimulating cleansing. Rotational exercises can assist relieve stress and have a significant balancing impact on our systems. Blockages are removed, and our energy can flow again.

Steps:

1. Stand with your feet shoulder-width apart and your arms out to the side, shoulder height.
2. Keep your torso steady and gradually begin to spin your body back and forth from right to left.
3. Repeat 5 to 10 times.

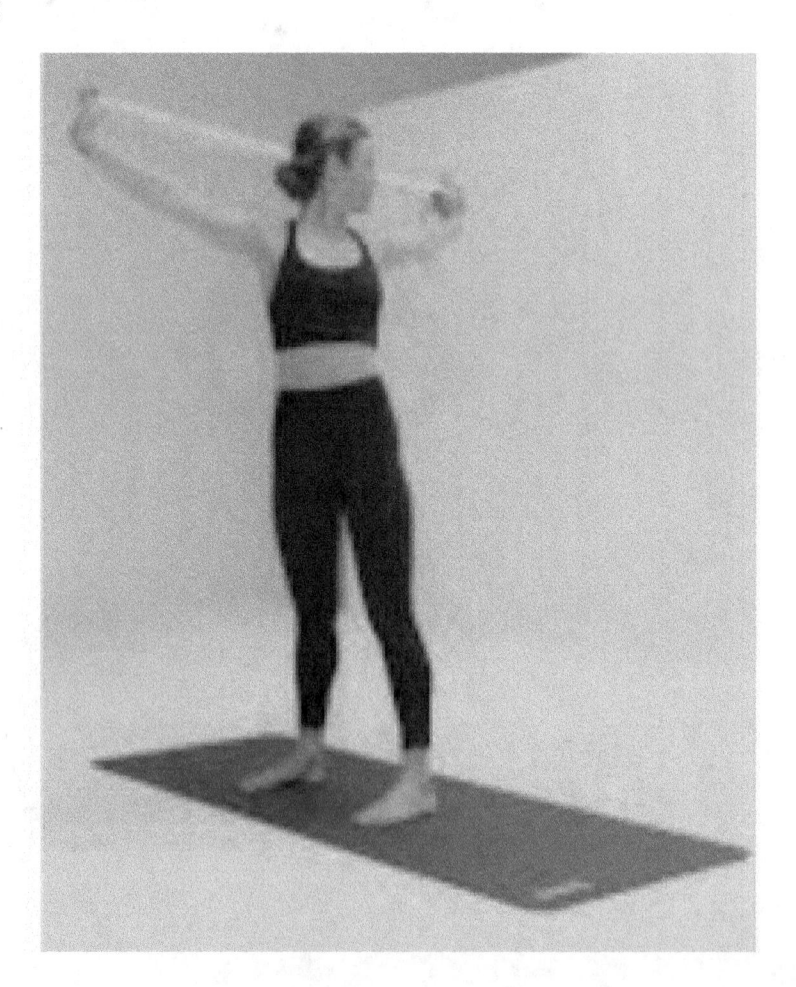

Illustration:

Day 21: **Rest & Reflection (Free Day)** **TIME: HOURS**

Engage in mindful movement throughout the day, such as stretching, walking, dancing, or simply listening to your body. Consider your adventure thus far. Note any insights or observations.

Wrap it Up at the end of each week!

Day 22: Arm Swings   TIME: 30 MINUTES

Swinging the arms often activates the nerves, tendons, and muscles that surround the shoulder joint.

Steps:

1. Stand with your arms outstretched at shoulder height in front of you, palms facing down.
2. Walk forward while swinging both arms to the right, with your left arm in front of your chest and your right arm out to the side. When swinging your arms, try to keep your body straight and simply turn your shoulders.
3. Continue walking while reversing the direction of the swing to the opposing side.
4. Repeat 5 times per side.

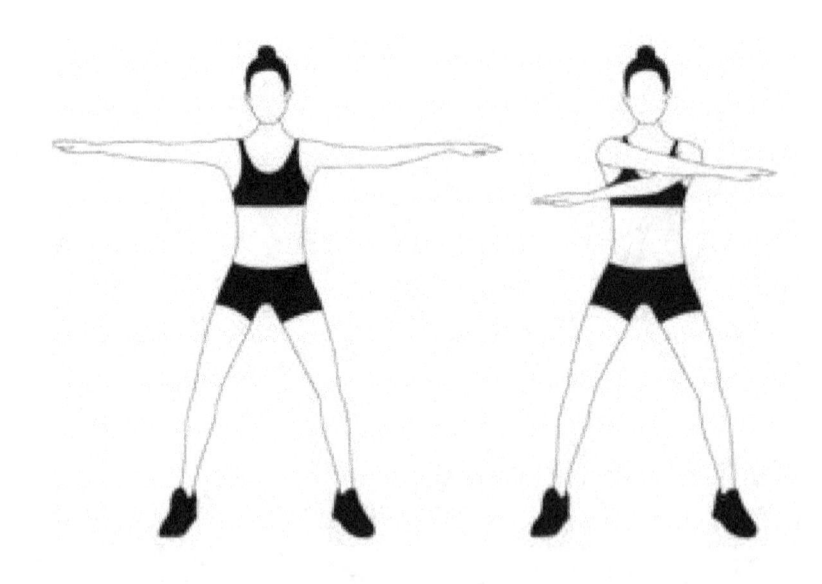

Illustration:

Day 23: Leg Pendulum TIME: 25 MINUTES

The heavy swinging also causes the muscles in our hips to relax, increasing oxygen flow down the legs.

Steps:

1. Begin swinging one leg back and forth while balancing on the other. If necessary, you can use a wall to support yourself.
2. Swing forwards and backwards 5-10 times.
3. Lower that leg and repeat with the other leg, swinging 5-10 times.
4. You may then face the wall and swing your legs from side to side if you like.

Illustration:

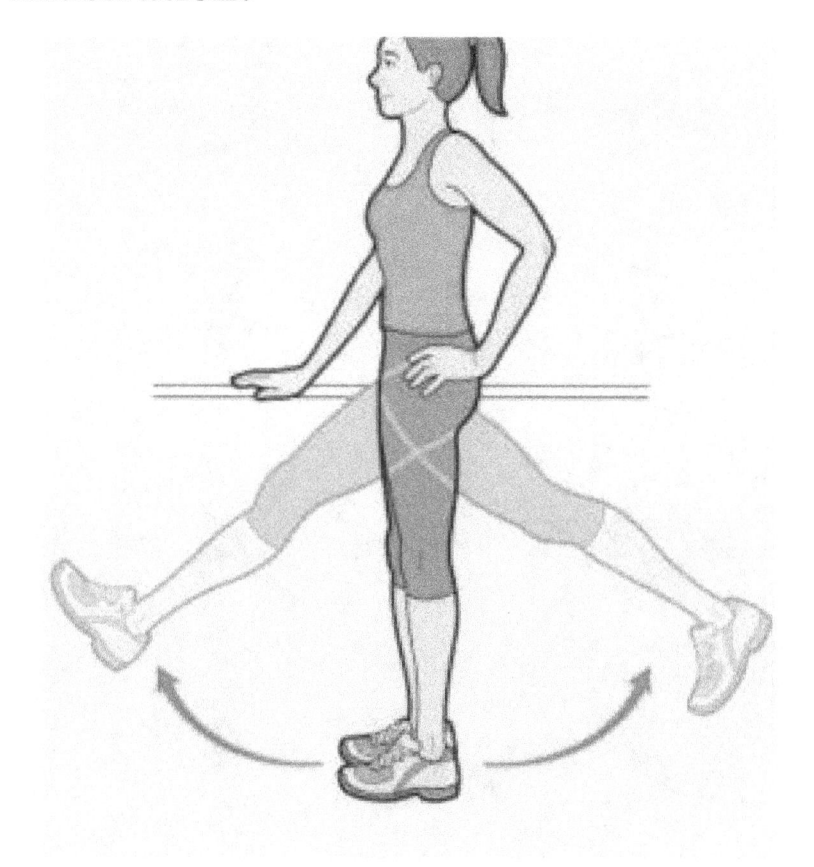

PRACTICE TO PERFECTION! KEEP GOING READER

Day 24: Hip and Pelvic Stability   TIME: 25 MINUTES

Pelvic stability training was reported to help improve trunk and lower extremity movement control, hip muscle strength, gait speed, and daily activities in stroke patients.

Steps:

1. Begin with a short body scan to identify any areas of stress.
2. Hip circles, pelvic tilts, and hip hinges are examples of exercises that focus on hip and pelvic stability.
3. Maintain a firm platform while you move your hips and pelvis through their complete range of motion.

Illustration:

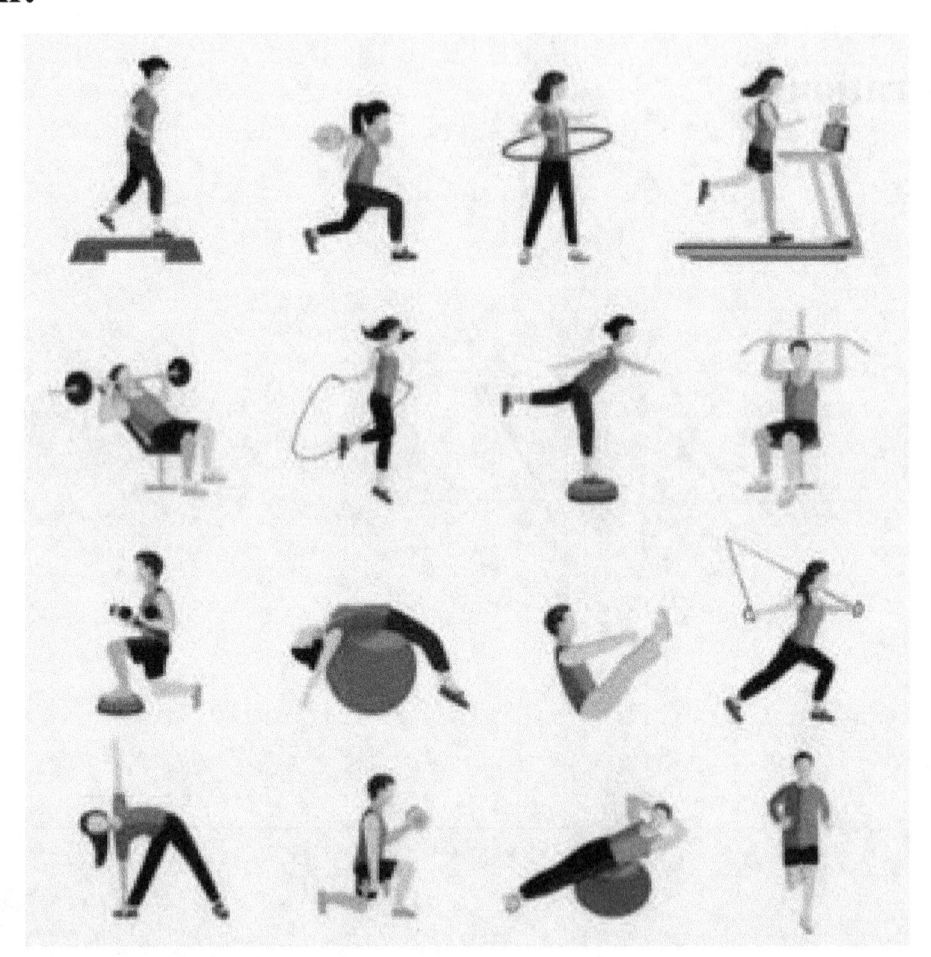

PRACTICE TO PERFECTION! KEEP GOING READER

Day 25: Mindful Walking   TIME: 30 MINUTES

Walking has physical advantages, but mindful walking can also lower blood pressure and heart rate, promote feelings of well-being, give better sleep, enhance mood, and manage stress.

Steps:

1. Begin with a brief sitting meditation centered on the breath.
2. Practice mindful walking by focusing on the feelings in your feet and legs as you move.
3. Concentrate on the rhythm of your steps and the relationship between your body and the surroundings.

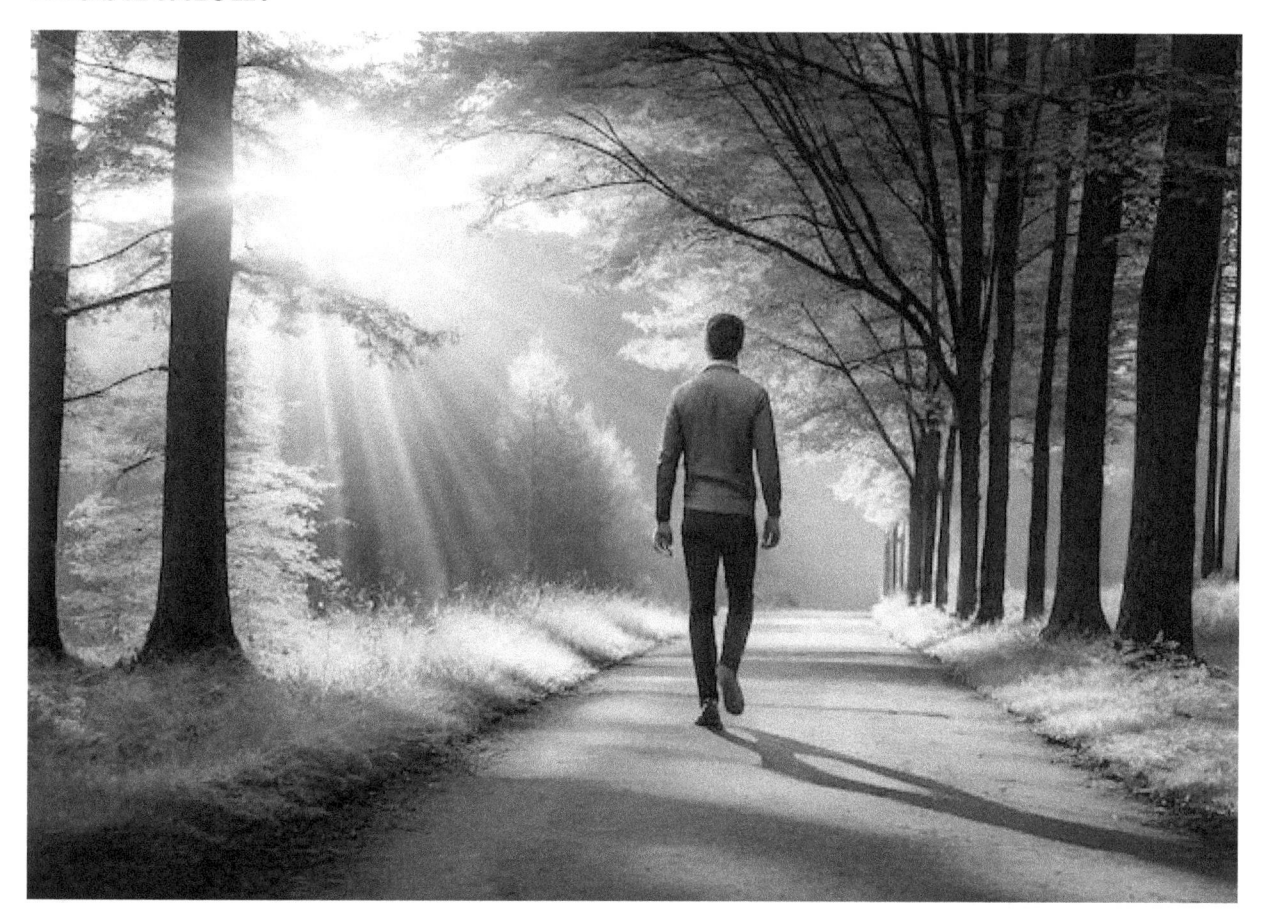

Illustration:

Day 26: Lower Body Awareness   TIME: 30 MINUTES

Body awareness is an important element of physical growth and can have a variety of benefits in our lives. It is critical to realize the importance of growing awareness since it may aid in the improvement of motor skills, physical performance, and self-confidence.

Steps:

1. Begin with deep breathing to calm the mind and body.

2. Perform lower-body exercises like hip circles and leg pendulums.

3. Concentrate on grounding and stability in the lower body, particularly the link between the feet and the ground.

Illustrations:

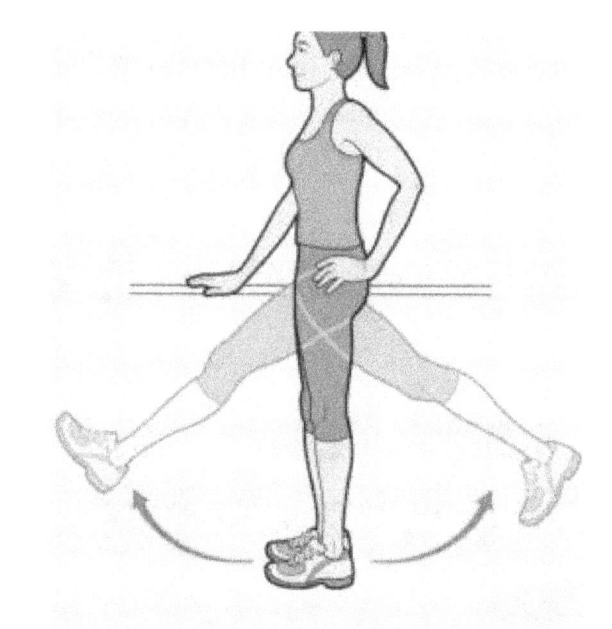

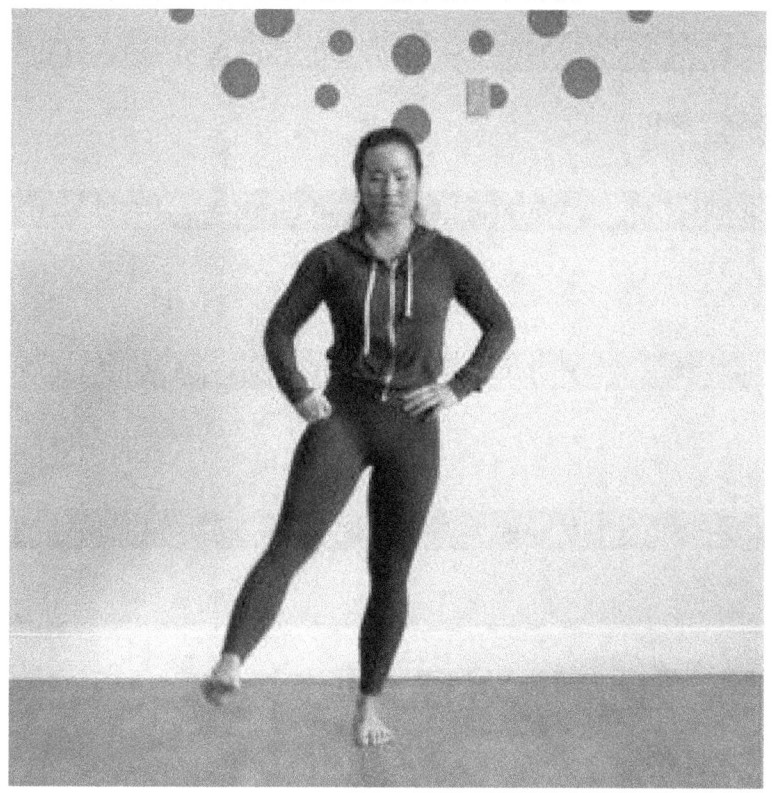

PRACTICE TO PERFECTION! KEEP GOING READER

Day 27: Modified Burpees   TIME: 30 MINUTES

Because even minimized burpees are a high-intensity workout, they burn more calories than walking, running, or using the elliptical at a slower pace. Improve your overall conditioning. You'll increase your heart rate and quickly acquire higher endurance.

Steps:

1. Begin by standing with your feet shoulder width apart and your arms by your sides.
2. Place your weight on your heels and drop yourself into a squat.
3. Stand back up, and instead of leaping like a normal burpee, stretch out to the sky while keeping your feet firmly on the ground.
4. Squat again, this time placing your hands flat on the ground immediately in front of you, moving your weight to them.
5. Instead of springing back into a plank posture like a conventional burpee, step your feet back one at a time.
6. Instead of executing a standard pushup, drop your knees to the ground and do a modified pushup.
7. Next, elevate your knees off the ground and rise onto your toes to form a plank position.
8. Walk your feet forward, one at a time, keeping your knees bent.
9. Stand up tall and grasp toward the sky.
10. Repeat. Build up your stamina by doing as many sets of modified burpees as possible.

Illustration:

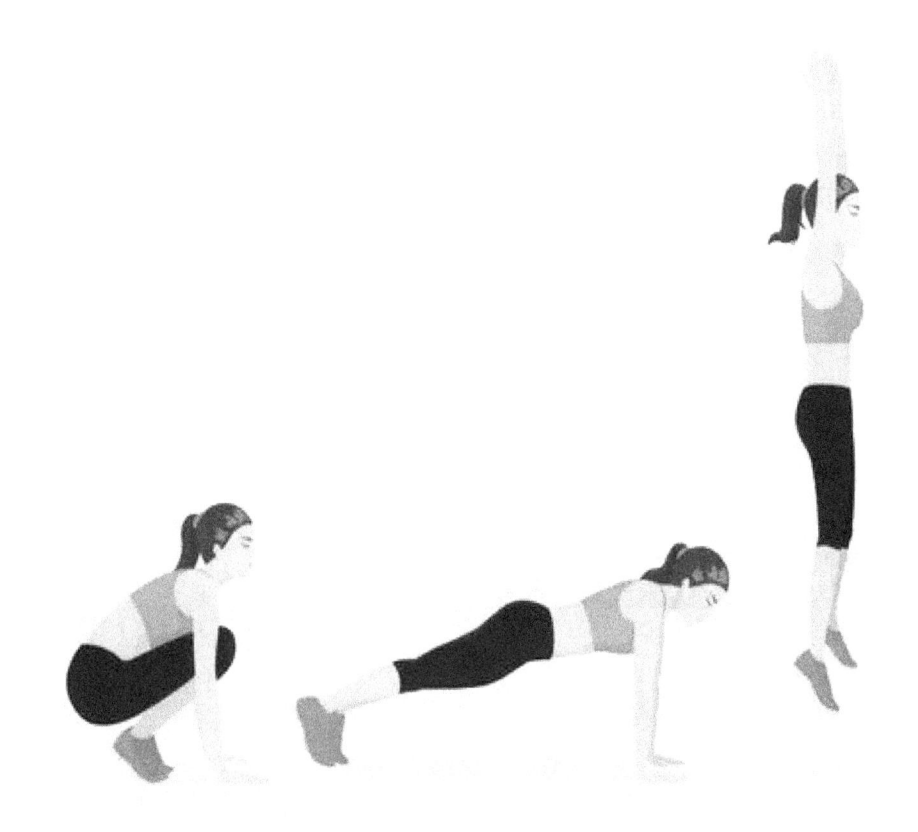

PRACTICE TO PERFECTION! KEEP GOING READER

Day 28: **Rest & Reflection** **TIME: 60 MINUTES**

- Take a day off to reflect on your development and experiences with somatic practice.
- Spend a few minutes in peaceful introspection or meditation, expressing thanks for your body and its talents.
- Use this opportunity to create goals for the following week of practice.

Wrap it Up at the end of each week!

Day 29: Chest Opening — TIME: 30 MINUTES

Opening the chest expands the front of the body, particularly the heart and lungs. This exercises the supplementary breathing muscles. Improved oxygen intake invigorates the body, stimulates cell metabolism, and improves focus.

Steps:

1. Stand or sit tall.
2. Hold both arms in front of you, palms together.
3. Inhale deeply, then bring your arms out and back.
4. Take several deep, cleansing breaths, and feel your chest and shoulders expand.
5. Squeeze your shoulder blades together while breathing.
6. Return both arms to the front, then repeat 5-10 times.

Illustration:

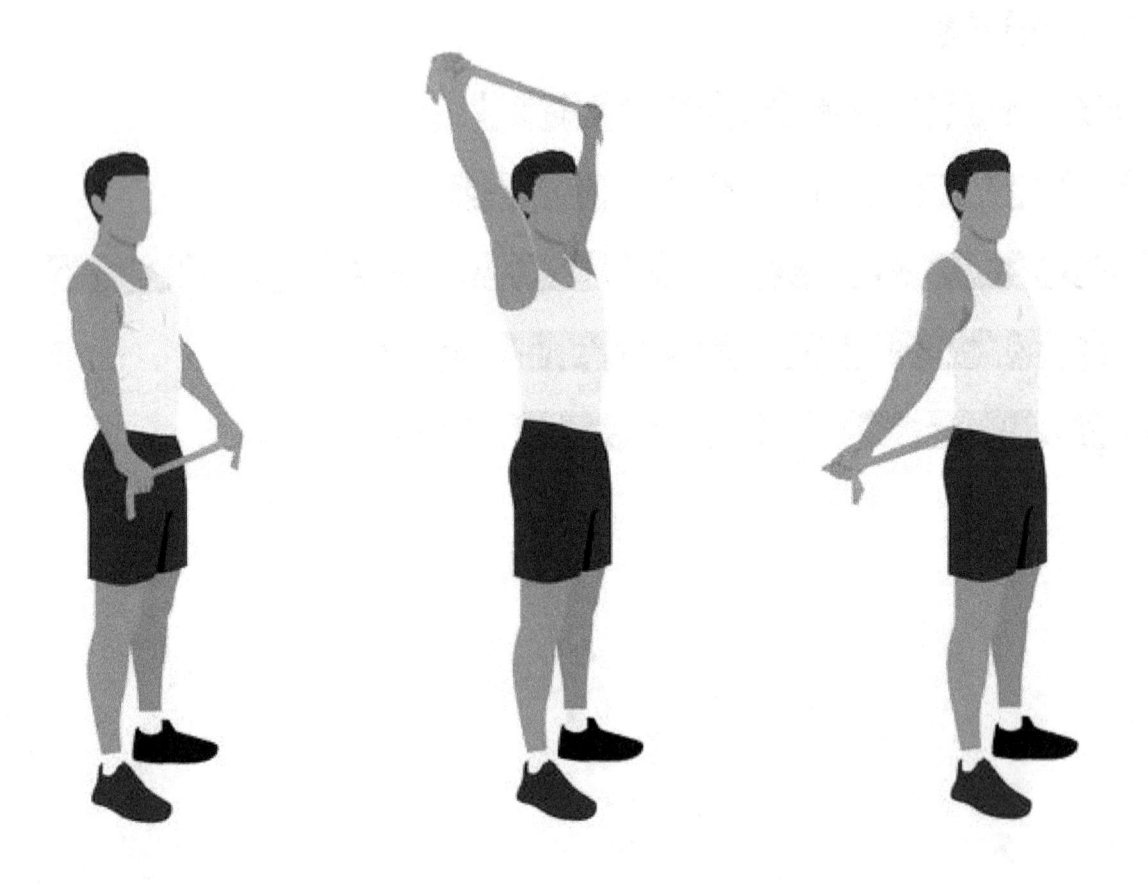

PRACTICE TO PERFECTION! KEEP GOING READER

Day 30: Baby Stretch   TIME: 30 MINUTES

Baby activities improve body awareness, strength, muscular tone, range of motion, and balance.

Steps:

1. Get to your hands and knees on the mat.
2. Spread your knees as wide as your mat, with the tops of your feet on the floor and the big toes touching.
3. Rest your tummy between your thighs and place your forehead on the floor. Relax your shoulders, jawline, and eyes. If placing the forehead on the floor is uncomfortable, try resting it on a block or two stacked fists.
4. Stretch your arms in front of you, palms facing the floor, or bring them back alongside your thighs, palms facing up.
5. Stay as long as you like, gradually reconnecting with the consistent inhales and exhales of your breath.

Illustration:

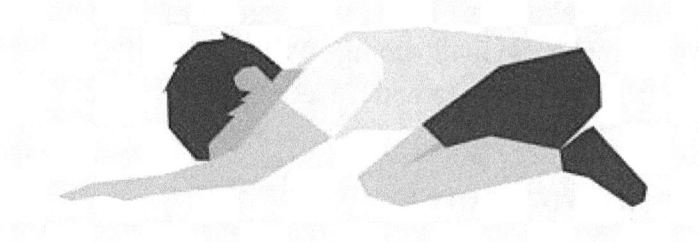

PRACTICE TO PERFECTION! KEEP GOING READER

Chapter 8: Somatic Workouts

In this chapter, we will look at somatic workouts, which integrate the concepts of somatic practice with typical fitness regimens. These workouts aim to increase body awareness, movement efficiency, and general well-being. Whether you're new to somatics or a seasoned practitioner, these routines provide a comprehensive approach to fitness that combines mind, body, and breath.

Overview of Somatic Workouts

Somatic exercises combine somatic concepts with components of strength, flexibility, and aerobic exercise. They emphasize attentive movement, breath synchronization, and body awareness to improve performance and lower the chance of injury. These workouts may be modified to specific requirements and fitness levels, making them suitable for a wide range of people.

Key Elements of Somatic Workouts;

1. *Thoughtful Warm-up*: Somatic exercises begin with a thoughtful warm-up that includes deep, diaphragmatic breathing and gentle movements to prepare the body for activity. This phase helps to calm the mind, raise body awareness, and relieve stress.

2. *Functional movement patterns*: Somatic exercises focus on functional movement patterns that are similar to those used in everyday activities. These exercises aim to increase mobility, stability, and coordination, hence increasing total movement efficiency.

3. *Breathe Integration*: Breath is included into every action in a somatic workout, strengthening the mind-body connection and encouraging relaxation. Coordinating breath and movement improves oxygenation, reduces stress, and increases endurance.

4. Progressive challenges: Somatic workouts test the body at escalating levels of intensity. This progressive approach allows for ongoing gains in strength, flexibility, and general fitness.

5. Cool down and relax: Somatic workouts culminate with a cool-down period that involves moderate stretching and relaxation techniques. This phase reduces muscular tension, promotes healing, and improves flexibility.

Benefits of Somatic Workout

- Improved Body Awareness: Somatic workouts improve body awareness by allowing people to listen into their bodies' signals and adapt their motions accordingly.

- Enhanced Movement Efficiency: Because somatic exercises focus on functional movement patterns, they reduce the chance of injury while also improving overall performance.

- Stress Reduction: The attentive aspect of somatic exercises promotes relaxation and decreases stress, resulting in a higher level of well-being.

- Improved Flexibility and Mobility: Somatic workouts increase flexibility and mobility, resulting in a wider range of motion and higher movement quality.

Sample Somatic Workout Routine

1. Warm-up (5 min): To focus the mind, begin by breathing deeply and diaphragmatically. To loosen up your body, try moderate motions like neck rolls, shoulder shrugs, and hip circles.

2. Strength Training (20 Minutes): Include functional strength exercises like squats, lunges, push-ups, and planks. Concentrate on good technique, breathing rhythm, and body alignment.

3. Cardiovascular Exercise (15 Minutes): Select a cardiovascular exercise you love, such as brisk walking, running, cycling, or dancing. Pay attention to your breathing and body feelings as you move.

4. Flexibility and Mobility (10 min): Include stretching exercises for important muscular groups such the hamstrings, quadriceps, calves, chest, shoulders, and back. Hold each stretch for 15-30 seconds, breathing deeply into it.

5. Cool down and relax (5 minutes): Finish with a gradual cool-down that incorporates slow, deep breathing and relaxing techniques. Concentrate on eliminating any leftover tension in the body and relaxing the thoughts.

Tips for Doing Somatic Workouts

- Start Slowly: If you're new to somatic training, begin with shorter sessions and progressively increase the time and intensity as you gain confidence.

- Listen to your body: Pay attention to how your body feels during the workout and change the intensity or tempo accordingly. Avoid pushing yourself over your boundaries.

- Remain Mindful: Throughout the workout, be careful of your breathing, body feelings, and movement patterns. This will help you remain present and attentive.

Integrating Somatics into Traditional Workouts

Traditional workouts are often designed to achieve external goals such as muscular growth, improved performance, or calorie burn. While these objectives are important, they sometimes miss the deeper link between your body and its inner workings. Here's where somatic practices come in. Somatics aims to improve interoception (internal awareness) and proprioception (body awareness), resulting in a more thoughtful and holistic approach to movement.

Advantages of Integrating Somatics:

- Enhanced Body Awareness: By focusing on subtle sensations and movement patterns, you can detect regions of tension, constriction, and imbalance. This awareness allows you to move more efficiently and reduces the danger of harm.
- Improved Form and Technique: Somatic concepts such as breathwork and alignment can improve your form in conventional exercises, resulting in more muscle engagement and better outcomes.
- Lowered Stress and Tension: Somatic practices frequently include mindfulness and gentle movements, which promote relaxation and reduce tension retained in the body, so improving healing and general well-being.
- Increased Movement Exploration: Integrating somatic activities like rolling, shaking, and fascial release broadens your movement vocabulary, resulting in a more diverse and pleasurable training experience.
- Deeper Connection to Your Body: Somatics fosters a deeper appreciation for your physical form and its capabilities, fostering a sense of embodiment and self-acceptance.

How To Integrate Somatics:

Begin with easy body scans: Before your workout, lie down for a few minutes and scan your body, noting any feelings without judgement. This creates the foundation for conscious movement.

Breathwork emphasis: Incorporate mindful breathing into your training routine. Coordinate your breathing with your movements, inhaling to expand and exhaling to relax. Coordinate your breath with your movements, using inhales to expand and exhales to release.

Pay attention to alignment and posture: Be conscious of your alignment throughout workouts, activating your core and maintaining good form. Concentrate on going from the center outwards.

Incorporate gentle stretches and releases: Add before a workout stretches and post-workout fascial release techniques using foam rollers or tennis balls to release tension and improve mobility.

Explore somatic movement practices: Think about adding short bursts of somatic exercises like yoga, tai chi, or Feldenkrais to your routine. These methods can improve your awareness and movement quality.

Listen to your body: Do not push yourself over your limits. Respect your body's signals and take pauses as required.

Example of integration:

Running: As you run, pay attention to the feelings in your feet, legs, and breathing. Instead, then focusing solely on speed, consider taking smooth, efficient steps.

Strength Training: When lifting weights, concentrate on connecting with the targeted muscle groups, feeling engagement and release with each action.

Yoga: Incorporate somatic concepts such as mindfulness and breathwork into your yoga practice to strengthen your connection with each position and its subtle sensations.

HIIT: During high-intensity exercise, utilize your breathing to control your effort and be present in your body. Listen to your signals and alter the intensity as necessary.

Creating Balanced Fitness Programs

Developing a balanced fitness program entails combining multiple training components to target different areas of physical health and well-being. A balanced program often incorporates aerobic activity, weight training, flexibility training, functional mobility, as well as rest and rehabilitation. The objective is to create a well-rounded regimen that improves overall fitness, lowers the chance of injury, and promotes long-term health and vitality.

Key Elements of a Balanced Fitness Program

1. Cardiovascular Exercise: This component aims to improve cardiovascular health, endurance, and stamina. Walking, jogging, cycling, swimming, and aerobic programs are typical ways to increase heart rate and enhance circulation.

2. Strength Training: Strength training consists of resistance exercises that improve muscle strength, endurance, and power. It promotes lean muscle mass, increases bone density, and improves overall body composition. Weightlifting, bodyweight exercises, resistance band workouts, and functional strength routines are all good examples.

3. Flexibility Training: Flexibility training aims to increase joint mobility, muscle elasticity, and range of motion. Stretching exercises, yoga, Pilates, and mobility drills are frequently used to maintain or improve flexibility while avoiding stiffness or injury.

4. Functional Movement: Functional movement training focuses on motions that simulate real-life tasks and improve daily functioning. It improves coordination, balance, and stability, all of which are necessary for everyday tasks and athletic performance. Squats, lunges, pushing, pulling, and rotating exercises are some examples.

5. Resting and Recovery: Adequate rest and recovery are required for the body to heal and adapt to the stresses of exercise. To encourage recovery and prevent overtraining, this component comprises rest days, adequate sleep, hydration, diet, and treatments such as foam rolling, massage, and relaxation exercises.

Principles for Developing a Balanced Fitness Program

- Individualization: Customize your program to meet your personal objectives, fitness level, and preferences. When developing your program, take into account age, fitness history, injuries, and lifestyle.

- Progress: Gradually increase the intensity, duration, or complexity of your exercises to keep your body challenged and prevent plateaus. This incremental strategy helps to prevent damage and promotes continuous improvement.

- Variation: Include a variety of workouts and activities to work different muscle groups, avoid boredom, and lower your chance of overuse problems. Change up your regimen with a variety of aerobic, weight training, and flexibility activities.

- Balance: Strive for a balance of different forms of exercise to avoid stressing one component of fitness at the expense of another. Incorporate aerobic and strength training, as well as flexibility and functional mobility, into your workout program.

- Recovery: Allow enough time for relaxation and recuperation in between sessions to avoid burnout and injury. Listen to your body's cues and alter your program accordingly to guarantee appropriate recuperation.

The Benefits of a Balanced Fitness Program

- Increased overall fitness: A well-balanced program covers all elements of fitness, resulting in improved cardiovascular health, muscle strength, flexibility, and functional mobility.

- Reduced Injury Risk: A balanced program that includes strength training, flexibility, and functional movement improves joint stability, muscle balance, and general body mechanics, lowering the risk of injury during exercise and daily activities.

- Enhanced Performance: A well-rounded program boosts athletic performance by increasing strength, endurance, agility, and coordination, all of which are necessary for sports and leisure activities.

- Improved health outcomes: Regular exercise, particularly when balanced and varied, can improve health outcomes, including a lower risk of chronic illnesses including heart disease, diabetes, and obesity.

Somatic Exercises for Beginners

Chapter 9: 30-Day Weight Loss Smoothies

DAY 1

Blackberry Smoothie

This blackberry smoothie is full of fresh fruit taste and sweetened with banana and honey. With only 5 minutes from start to finish, it's the ideal breakfast for a hectic morning. If fresh blackberries are not available, you may use frozen blackberries in this simple and nutritious smoothie.

Prep Time: 5 mins

Total Time: 5 mins

Servings: 1

Ingredients:

1 cup of fresh blackberries (6 ounces).

½ medium banana.

1/2 cup plain whole-milk Greek yogurt.

1 tablespoon honey.

1 ½ teaspoon fresh lemon juice.

1 teaspoon of freshly chopped fresh ginger.

Directions:

Blend together blackberries, banana, yogurt, honey, lemon juice, and ginger. Cover and process for approximately 2 minutes, or until fully smooth. Serve immediately.

Nutrition Value (per serving):

316	7g	53g	15g
Calories	Fat	Carbs	Protein

DAY 2

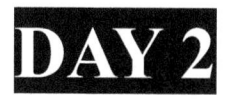

Strawberry-Banana Protein Smoothie

In this fresh fruit smoothie recipe, Greek yogurt and nut butter offer protein, while ground flaxseed adds omega-3s. If you want a chilly smoothie, use ice cubes, but if you don't, use water instead.

Prep Time: 10 mins

Total Time: 10 mins

Servings: 1

Ingredients:

1 cup hulled strawberries (fresh or frozen).

½ medium banana.

1/2 cup chopped mango, fresh or frozen.

1/2 cup nonfat plain Greek yogurt

1 tablespoon of natural nut butter, such cashew or almond.

1 tablespoon of ground flaxseed (flaxmeal).

¼ teaspoon vanilla extract.

Four ice cubes or one-half cup water

Directions:

In a blender, combine strawberries, banana, mango, yogurt, nut butter, flaxmeal, vanilla, and ice (or water). Puree till smooth

Nutrition Value (per serving):

359	14g	46g	19g
Calories	Fat	Carbs	Protein

DAY 3

Banana-Cocoa Soy Smoothie

With lots of protein from tofu and soymilk, this banana-split-inspired morning smoothie will keep you full until midday.

Prep Time: 5 mins

Total Time: 1 hr

Servings: 1

Ingredients:

1 banana.

1/2 cup silken tofu.

½ cup soy milk

2 tablespoons of unsweetened cocoa powder.

1 tablespoon honey.

Directions:

Slice the banana and freeze until solid. Blend the tofu, soymilk, chocolate, and honey in a blender until smooth. With the machine going, insert the banana slices through the hole in the cover and purée until smooth.

Nutrition Value (per serving):

342	8g	62g	16g
Calories	Fat	Carbs	Protein

DAY 4

Anti-Inflammatory Beet Smoothie

This vivid beet smoothie blends sweet and earthy beets with berries, banana, and orange juice for a well-balanced flavor. Look for packaged cooked beets at stores that sell prepared fruits and vegetables. Beets are high in belatins, an antioxidant that may aid to reduce inflammation in the body. Other nutrient-dense substances, such as anthocyanins in blueberries and gingerol in ginger, boost anti-inflammatory activity even more.

Prep Time: 5 mins

Total Time: 5 mins

Servings: 2

Ingredients:

1 cup frozen strawberries.

1 cup of frozen blueberries.

1 cup orange juice.

1 (8.8-ounce) bag of refrigerated cooked beets (such as Love Beets).

1 medium, peeled banana

One medium carrot, peeled and sliced

One (1/2 inch) piece of fresh ginger, peeled and grated

Directions:

In a blender, mix strawberries, blueberries, orange juice, beets, banana, carrot, and ginger. Process for about 30 seconds. Divide between two glasses. Serve immediately.

Nutrition Value (per serving):

248	1g	58g	4g
Calories	Fat	Carbs	Protein

DAY 5

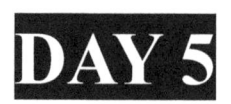

Cherry-Berry Oatmeal Smoothies

Add some oats to your fruit smoothie for extra staying power--this simple breakfast will keep you going all morning.

Prep Time: 10 mins

Total Time: 15 mins

Servings: 3

Ingredients:

½ cup water

⅓ cup quick-cook rolled oats

1/2 cup light almond or fat-free milk

¾ cup fresh or frozen unsweetened strawberries, partly thawed

½ cup fresh or frozen pitted dark delicious cherries, partly thawed

1–2 tbsp almond butter

1 tablespoon honey.

1/2 cup tiny ice cubes.

Directions:

Step 1: In a medium bowl, mix water and oats. Microwave for 1 minute. Stir in 1/4 cup of milk. Microwave for 30 to 50 seconds more, or until the oats are extremely soft. Cool for 5 minutes.

Step 2: In a blender, combine the oat mixture, 1/4 cup milk, and other four ingredients (through honey). Cover and mix until smooth, scraping the container as necessary. Add ice cubes, cover, and mix until smooth. If desired, top each dish with more fruit.

Nutrition Value (per serving):

121	4g	21g	3g
Calories	Fat	Carbs	Protein

DAY 6

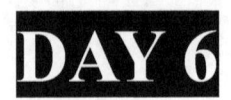

Strawberry-Chocolate Smoothie

This creamy, luscious strawberry-chocolate smoothie will fulfill all your chocolate desires. It's so decadent that you might even want it for dessert.

Prep Time: 5 mins

Total Time: 5 mins

Servings: 1

Ingredients:

1 1/2 cups frozen strawberries

1 cup of chilled chocolate-unsweetened almond milk, plus more as required.

1 tablespoon almond butter.

1 tablespoon of unsweetened cocoa powder.

1 tablespoon honey.

Directions:

In a blender, combine strawberries, almond milk, almond butter, chocolate, and honey. Blend until smooth, adding additional almond milk as required for the desired consistency. Serve immediately.

Nutrition Value (per serving):

303	13g	47g	7g
Calories	Fat	Carbs	Protein

DAY 7

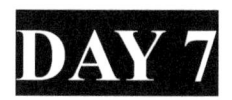

Ultimate Healthy Breakfast Smoothie

This nutritious morning smoothie recipe contains protein, fiber, unsaturated fats, and vital vitamins and minerals. Follow our easy procedure, remember the component proportions, and then tailor to your preferences. Even better, our supercharged morning smoothie is delicious and keeps you satisfied until midday. We keep frozen bananas on hand to thicken our smoothies, but a handful of ice works just as well.

Prep Time: 5 mins

Total Time: 5 mins

Servings: 1

Ingredients:

1 medium banana, fresh or frozen.

1/2 cup sliced strawberries, blueberries, or diced mangos.

1/4 cup plain 2% Greek yogurt.

1 tablespoon almond butter

1/2 cup baby spinach

1/2 cup unsweetened almond milk.

1-2 basil leaves, 2-3 mint leaves, or 1/2 teaspoon peeled and diced ginger (optional).

Directions:

In a blender, combine banana, strawberries (or blueberries or mango), yogurt, almond butter, spinach, almond milk, and basil (or mint or ginger, if using). Process until smooth.

Tips: If the smoothie is too thick, add an extra dash of almond milk. If the smoothie is too thin, thicken it with a handful of ice.

To make a dairy-free smoothie, replace Greek yogurt with coconut milk yogurt. For a nut-free smoothie, use ground flax seeds, sunflower seeds, or pumpkin seeds instead of almond butter.

Nutrition Value (per serving):

300	11g	40g	13g
Calories	Fat	Carbs	Protein

DAY 8

Chocolate-Banana Protein Smoothie

The red lentils in this smoothie provide a plant-based protein boost. To make this smoothie vegan, substitute unsweetened coconut or almond milk for the dairy milk.

Prep Time: 5 mins

Total Time: 5 mins

Servings: 1

Ingredients:

One banana, frozen

1/2 cup cooked red lentils.

½ cup nonfat milk.

2 tablespoons of unsweetened cocoa powder.

1 teaspoon of pure maple syrup.

Directions:

In a blender, combine the banana, lentils, milk, chocolate, and syrup. Puree till smooth.

Nutrition Value (per serving):

310	2g	64g	15g
Calories	Fat	Carbs	Protein

DAY 9

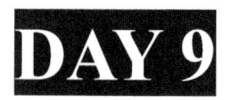

Grape Smoothie

Calling all grape lovers! This grape smoothie has a lot of frozen sweet red grapes mixed with banana and vanilla Greek-style yogurt, both of which contribute smoothness, while berries offer color and delicious flavor to match the grapes.

Prep Time:	*Total Time:*	*Servings:*
15 mins	4 hrs 15 mins	2

Ingredients:

3 cups seedless red grapes (plus extra for garnish)

1 cup strawberries, stems and halved.

¾ cup fresh blueberries

1/2 medium banana, peeled and sliced.

⅓ cup vanilla strained Greek-style yogurt made from whole milk

¼ cup water

⅛ teaspoon kosher salt.

Directions:

Step 1: Wash and dry the grapes thoroughly with paper towels. Spread in an equal layer on a large rimmed baking sheet coated with parchment paper. Freeze for approximately 4 hours, or until absolutely hard.

Step 2: In a blender, combine the frozen grapes, strawberries, blueberries, banana, yogurt, water, and salt. Blend until totally smooth, about 1 minute, stopping to scrape down the sides and stir as needed. Pour into two big glasses. If desired, garnish each smoothie with three grapes tied onto a wooden pick. Serve immediately.

Nutrition Value (per serving):

282	2g	66g	6g
Calories	Fat	Carbs	Protein

DAY 10

Pineapple Green Smoothie

Use ripe bananas to make this creamy Greek yogurt, spinach, and pineapple smoothie. Chia seeds include healthful omega-3 fats, fiber, and a little amount of protein, providing an added nutritious boost.

Prep Time:	*Total Time:*	*Servings:*
5 mins	5 mins	1

Ingredients:

1/2 cup unsweetened almond milk.

⅓ cup nonfat plain Greek yogurt

1 cup baby spinach.

1 cup frozen banana slices (about one medium banana

1/2 cup frozen pineapple chunks.

1 tablespoon of chia seeds.

1-2 tablespoons of pure maple syrup or honey (optional).

Directions:

In a blender, combine almond milk and yogurt, then add spinach, banana, pineapple, chia seeds, and sweetener (if using). Blend until smooth.

Nutrition Value (per serving):

297	6g	54g	13g
Calories	Fat	Carbs	Protein

DAY 11

Strawberry-Blueberry-Banana Smoothie

A smoothie made with strawberries, blueberries, and banana is gently sweet and completely kid-friendly, even with the added protein from hemp seeds. Freeze the fruits ahead of time to achieve an additional icy texture when combined.

Prep Time:	Total Time:	Servings:
5 mins	5 mins	1

Ingredients:

½ cup frozen strawberries.

½ cup frozen blueberries.

One tiny ripe banana (frozen if preferred)

¾ cup cold unsweetened cashew milk, plus more as required.

1 tablespoon of cashew butter.

1 tablespoon of hulled hemp seeds.

Directions:

Mix strawberries, blueberries, banana, cashew milk, cashew butter, and hemp seeds in a blender. Process until smooth, adding additional cashew milk as required to get the desired consistency. Serve immediately.

Nutrition Value (per serving):

335	17g	46g	7g
Calories	Fat	Carbs	Protein

DAY 12

Fruit & Yogurt Smoothie

This simple fruit smoothie recipe calls for only three ingredients: yogurt, fruit juice, and frozen fruits. Change up your fruit combinations every day for a nutritious breakfast or snack that never gets dull.

Prep Time: 10 mins

Total Time: 10 mins

Servings: 1

Ingredients:

3/4 cup nonfat plain yogurt.

1/2 cup 100% pure fruit juice.

1 1/2 cups (6 1/2 ounces) of frozen fruit, like blueberries, raspberries, pineapple, or peaches

Directions:

Blend yogurt and juice until smooth. While the machine is working, pour the fruit through the hole in the cover and puree until smooth.

Nutrition Value (per serving):

279	2g	56g	12g
Calories	Fat	Carbs	Protein

DAY 13

Spinach-Avocado Smoothie

The frozen banana and avocado make this healthy green smoothie extra creamy. Make ahead (up to one day) and refrigerate until you need a vegetable boost.

Prep Time: 5 mins

Total Time: 5 mins

Servings: 1

Ingredients:

One cup of nonfat plain yogurt

1 cup of fresh spinach.

One frozen banana.

¼ Avocado

2 tablespoons of water.

1 teaspoon honey.

Directions:

Blend yogurt, spinach, banana, avocado, water, and honey in a blender. Puree till smooth.

Nutrition Value (per serving):

357	8g	58g	18g
Calories	Fat	Carbs	Protein

DAY 14

Carrot-Apple Smoothie

This carrot and apple smoothie is creamy and has a subtle tropical taste from coconut milk. The carrots and apple naturally sweeten it, while the ginger and lemon juice combo offer a hint of spiciness while also helping to balance the flavor. Turmeric, whether fresh or dried, gives the smoothie a rich orange hue.

Prep Time: 5 mins

Total Time: 5 mins

Servings: 2

Ingredients:

2 big carrots, cut (about. 1 1/2 cups).

1 medium ripe banana.

One big Honeycrisp apple, cored and quartered

1 cup of light coconut milk.

2 teaspoons of fresh lemon juice.

2 tsp minced fresh ginger

2 tsp chopped fresh turmeric or 1 tsp ground turmeric

1/2 cup ice cubes.

Directions:

In a blender, combine carrots, bananas, apples, coconut milk, lemon juice, ginger, and turmeric. Process for approximately 45 seconds, or until smooth. Process in ice cubes until smooth, about 30 seconds. Serve immediately.

Nutrition Value (per serving):

243	8g	46g	4g
Calories	Fat	Carbs	Protein

DAY 15

Passion Fruit Smoothie

This three-ingredient smoothie contains frozen passion fruit, which has strong floral aromas and a tangy taste. While any sort of kiwi will work, we prefer yellow kiwi since it gives more taste, natural sweetness, and improves the color. Taste and finish with a spoonful or two of honey to balance the flavors.

Prep Time: 5 mins

Total Time: 5 mins

Servings: 1

Ingredients:

1 cup frozen passion fruit.

One kiwi, peeled

1/2 cup reduced-fat or unsweetened nondairy milk

1–2 tablespoons honey (optional)

Directions:

In a blender, combine passion fruit, kiwi, milk, and honey to taste (if using). Process on high until extremely smooth.

Nutrition Value (per serving):

252	4g	52g	8g
Calories	Fat	Carbs	Protein

DAY 16

Cherry-Mocha Smoothie

Make a quick breakfast on the run with your blender. The beneficial fats in the almond butter, as well as the health-boosting phytonutrients in the cocoa powder and cherries in this delicious morning smoothie, protect against heart disease.

Prep Time:
10 mins

Total Time:
10 mins

Servings:
2

Ingredients:

1 cup frozen unsweetened pitted dark delicious cherries.

1 cup of unsweetened chocolate almond milk.

5.3 to 6-ounce container of vanilla fat-free Greek yogurt.

½ medium banana (see Tip).

2 tablespoons of unsweetened cocoa powder.

2 tablespoons almond butter.

1 teaspoon of instant espresso coffee powder.

1 teaspoon vanilla.

Two cups of ice cubes

1 tablespoon dark chocolate shavings and chocolate-covered espresso beans

Directions:

In a blender, add cherries, almond milk, Greek yogurt, banana, chocolate powder, almond butter, espresso coffee powder, and vanilla. Cover and mix until smooth. Add ice cubes, cover, and mix until smooth. Pour into glasses, and if desired, garnish with chocolate shavings, chocolate-covered espresso beans, and/or extra banana slices (see Tip).

Tips: Peel the remaining banana half and cover it securely in plastic wrap, then in foil. Freeze for later use. Alternatively, divide the ice cubes between two tall glasses rather than mixing them with the smoothie. To serve, pour the smoothie over the ice cubes.

Nutrition Value (per serving):

272	12g	34g	13g
Calories	Fat	Carbs	Protein

DAY 17

Berry-Kefir Smoothie

When you add kefir to your smoothie for morning, it provides a probiotic boost. Feel free to use any fruit and nut butter you have on hand for this nutritious smoothie recipe.

Prep Time: 5 mins

Total Time: 5 mins

Servings: 1

Ingredients:

1 1/2 cups frozen mixed berries

1 cup plain kefir.

½ medium banana.

2 teaspoons almond butter.

½ teaspoon vanilla extract.

Directions:

Blend berries, kefir, banana, almond butter, and vanilla in a blender. Blend until smooth.

Nutrition Value (per serving):

304	7g	53g	15g
Calories	Fat	Carbs	Protein

DAY 18

Avocado & Banana Smoothie

If you enjoy creamy smoothies, this one is for you: avocado and banana mix to create a thick and rich drink. Freeze the banana slices to make it more like an ice cream smoothie.

Prep Time: 10 mins

Total Time: 10 mins

Servings: 1

Ingredients:

Ingredients: 1 medium sliced banana and 1/2 pitted and sliced avocado.

2 teaspoons honey.

5–6 ice cubes

⅔ cup unsweetened vanilla almond or coconut milk

Directions:

Step 1: Blend together the banana, avocado, honey, ice cubes, and coconut milk (or almond milk). Blend on medium-low speed, using the tamper if needed, until well blended.

Step 2: Increase the speed to medium-high, and mix until extremely smooth.

Nutrition Value (per serving):

338	18g	48g	3g
Calories	Fat	Carbs	Protein

DAY 19

Strawberry-Mango-Banana Smoothie

Making fruit smoothies at home saves both time and money. For this simple smoothie, mix strawberries, mango, and banana with cashew butter and powdered chia seeds for body and richness.

Prep Time: 5 mins

Total Time: 5 mins

Servings: 1

Ingredients:

½ cup frozen strawberries.

1/2 cup diced ripe mango.

1/2 medium-ripe banana (frozen if preferred)

½ cup unsweetened refrigerated coconut milk beverage (e.g., So Delicious), or more as required.

1 tablespoon of cashew butter.

1 tablespoon of ground chia seeds.

Directions:

Mix strawberries, mango, banana, coconut milk, cashew butter, and chia seeds in a blender. Process until smooth, adding additional coconut milk as required to get the desired consistency. Serve immediately.

Nutrition Value (per serving):

299	15g	42g	5g
Calories	Fat	Carbs	Protein

DAY 20

Thermos-Ready Smoothie

This nutritious smoothie recipe provides a protein and fiber-rich drink on the run.

Prep Time: 5 mins

Total Time: 5 mins

Servings: 1

Ingredients:

1 cup frozen mixed berries.

½ banana

1/2 cup apple juice.

¼ cup silken tofu

Directions:

In a blender, combine the berries, banana, apple juice, and tofu. Blend until smooth.

Nutrition Value (per serving):

276	3g	62g	6g
Calories	Fat	Carbs	Protein

DAY 21

Creamsicle Breakfast Smoothie

Though it tastes like the legendary vanilla-and-orange popsicles, this creamsicle morning smoothie recipe is a well-balanced meal rich in carbs, protein, and, due to the inclusion of coconut water, electrolytes. Coconut water has more than 10% of your daily potassium requirement--an electrolyte lost via sweat--in every cup, making it an excellent hydrator for mild exercises. Furthermore, this creamy orange-mango smoothie includes just approximately 30 mg of sodium per cup, whereas sports drinks typically have 110 mg of salt per cup.

Prep Time: 5 mins

Total Time: 5 mins

Servings: 2

Ingredients:

1 cup chilled, pure coconut water with no additional sugar or taste (see Tip)

1 cup of nonfat vanilla Greek yogurt.

1 cup of frozen or fresh mango pieces.

3 tablespoons of frozen orange juice concentrate.

Two cups of ice

Directions:

Blend the coconut water, yogurt, mango, orange juice concentrate, and ice in a blender until smooth.

Tips: Look for pure coconut water without additional sugar in the refrigerated section, amid flavored waters, shelf-stable fluids, and natural fruit juices.

Nutrition Value (per serving):

184	1g	33g	13g
Calories	Fat	Carbs	Protein

DAY 22

Berry-Coconut Smoothie

Lentils may provide protein and fiber to your smoothie without the use of dairy or protein powder. They're a secret source of plant-based protein in this nutritious smoothie recipe.

Prep Time:	*Total Time:*	*Servings:*
10 mins	10 mins	1

Ingredients:

½ cup cooked and cooled red lentils (see Tips).

¾ cup unsweetened vanilla coconut milk drink

1/2 cup frozen mixed berries.

1/2 cup frozen sliced banana.

1 tablespoon unsweetened shredded coconut, with more for garnish.

1 teaspoon honey and 2 ice cubes.

Directions:

Combine lentils, coconut milk, berries, banana, coconut, honey, and ice cubes in a blender. Blend on high for 2-3 minutes, or until extremely smooth. If desired, add extra coconut as garnish.

<u>*Tips*</u> for cooking red lentils: Cook in boiling water for approximately 15 minutes, or until just tender. Drain and chill. 1 cup dry equals 2 1/2 cups cooked. Refrigerate for up to three days. Alternatively, freeze in 1/2-cup quantities for up to three months (thaw before use).

Nutrition Value (per serving):

322	8g	58g	11g
Calories	Fat	Carbs	Protein

DAY 23

Pumpkin Pie Smoothie

This healthy smoothie recipe has the same flavor of a pumpkin spice latte but without the added sugar. Made with genuine pumpkin and frozen banana, this creamy, delectable grab-and-go breakfast (or snack) takes only 5 minutes to prepare.

Prep Time: 5 mins

Total Time: 5 mins

Servings: 1

Ingredients:

One medium frozen banana.

1/2 cup unsweetened almond milk (or other nut milk).

⅓ cup plain whole milk Greek yogurt

⅓ cup canned pumpkin puree.

⅛ teaspoon Pumpkin Pie Spice

1-2 tablespoons of pure maple syrup.

Directions:

Combine the banana, almond milk (or other nut milk), yogurt, pumpkin puree, pumpkin pie spice, and maple syrup in a blender. Blend until smooth.

Nutrition Value (per serving):

247	6g	42g	10g
Calories	Fat	Carbs	Protein

DAY 24

Peanut Butter-Strawberry-Kale Smoothie

This PB&J-inspired green smoothie recipe is ideal for a quick and nutritious breakfast on the road.

Prep Time: 5 mins

Total Time: 5 mins

Servings: 1

Ingredients:

- 1 cup unsweetened soymilk
- 1 cup frozen strawberries.
- 1 cup chopped Kal.
- 1 tablespoon of natural peanut butter.
- 1 tablespoon honey.
- 1 teaspoon of vanilla essence.
- 2–4 ice cubes

Directions:

Blend soymilk, strawberries, kale, peanut butter, honey, vanilla, and ice cubes in a blender. Puree till smooth.

Nutrition Value (per serving):

321	12g	40g	12g
Calories	Fat	Carbs	Protein

DAY 25

Mango-Ginger Smoothie

Red lentils are an unexpected source of plant-based protein in this nutritious smoothie recipe. The lentils provide 3 grams more protein than an equal-sized serving of nonfat plain yogurt and 4 grams more fiber than a standard serving of protein powder.

Prep Time: 10 mins

Total Time: 10 mins

Servings: 1

Ingredients:

½ cup cooked and cooled red lentils (see Tips).

1 cup of frozen mango chunks.

¾ cup carrot juice

1 teaspoon chopped fresh ginger

1 teaspoon honey.

A pinch of ground cardamom, plus more for garnish.

Three ice cubes.

Directions:

Combine lentils, mango, carrot juice, ginger, honey, cardamom, and ice cubes in a blender. Blend on high for 2-3 minutes, or until extremely smooth. Garnish with additional cardamom if desired.

<u>*Tips*</u> for cooking red lentils: Cook in boiling water for approximately 15 minutes, or until just tender. Drain and chill. 1 cup dry equals 2 1/2 cups cooked. Refrigerate for up to three days. Alternatively, freeze in 1/2-cup quantities for up to three months (thaw before use).

Nutrition Value (per serving):

352	1g	79g	12g
Calories	Fat	Carbs	Protein

DAY 26

Blueberry-Cranberry Smoothie

Are you ready to try kefir? We use it instead of yogurt in this healthy smoothie recipe with berries and bananas.

Prep Time:

5 mins

Total Time:

5 mins

Servings:

1

Ingredients:

½ frozen medium banana.

1 cup of frozen blueberries.

½ cup frozen cranberries.

1 cup low-fat plain kefir.

Directions:

Blend banana, blueberries, cranberries, and kefir in a blender. Puree till smooth.

Nutrition Value (per serving):

245	1g	50g	13g
Calories	Fat	Carbs	Protein

DAY 27

Cantaloupe Smoothie

This nutritious smoothie recipe is ideal for cooling down in the summer when cantaloupes are at their optimum, bringing lots of sweetness to this healthy snack.

Prep Time: 10 mins

Total Time: 10 mins

Servings: 1

Ingredients:

1 banana.

2 cups diced, ripe cantaloupe

1/2 cup nonfat or low-fat plain yogurt

2 teaspoons of nonfat dry milk.

1 ½ teaspoons frozen orange juice concentrate.

½ teaspoon vanilla extract.

Directions: Step 1: Put the unpeeled banana in the freezer overnight (or for up to three months).

Step 2: Take the banana out of the freezer and let it sit for approximately 2 minutes, or until the peel softens. Use a paring knife to remove the skin. (Don't worry if any fiber remains.) Cut the banana into bits. Add to a blender or food processor with the cantaloupe, yogurt, dry milk, orange juice, and vanilla. Blend until smooth.

Tips: Make Ahead Tip: Freeze the banana for up to three months.

Nutrition Value (per serving):

364	3g	75g	14g
Calories	Fat	Carbs	Protein

DAY 28

Strawberry-Pineapple Smoothie

Blend almond milk, strawberry, and pineapple for a simple smoothie that you can make on a busy morning. A spoonful of almond butter provides richness and satisfying protein. Freeze portion of the almond milk to achieve an extra-icy texture.

Prep Time: 5 mins

Total Time: 5 mins

Servings: 1

Ingredients:

1 cup frozen strawberries.

1 cup of chopped fresh pineapple.

¾ cup cold unsweetened almond milk, plus more as required.

1 tablespoon almond butter.

Directions:

Mix strawberries, pineapple, almond milk, and almond butter in a blender. Process until smooth, adding additional almond milk as required to get the desired consistency. Serve immediately.

Nutrition Value (per serving):

255	11g	39g	6g
Calories	Fat	Carbs	Protein

DAY 29

Jason Mraz's Avocado Green Smoothie

Mraz, the singer, adds a spoonful of coconut oil and some sprouted flax or chia seeds to this green smoothie recipe to turn it into a meal in a glass.

Prep Time: 15 mins

Total Time: 15 mins

Servings: 2

Ingredients:

1 ¼ cups chilled, unsweetened almond or coconut milk beverage

1 ripe avocado.

One ripe banana.

Ingredients: 1 sliced Honeycrisp apple and 1/2 big or 1 small celery stalk, diced.

2 cups of lightly packed kale leaves or spinach

1 1-inch piece of peeled fresh ginger.

Eight ice cubes.

Directions:

Blend the milk beverage, avocado, banana, apple, celery, kale (or spinach), ginger, and ice until smooth.

Nutrition Value (per serving):

307	17g	40g	5g
Calories	Fat	Carbs	Protein

DAY 30

Mango Raspberry Smoothie

A dash of lemon juice brightens the flavor of this frozen fruit smoothie. Mango gives enough of sweetness without the need for juice, but if it's too sour, a bit of agave can help.

Prep Time: 5 mins

Total Time: 5 mins

Servings: 1

Ingredients:

Add ½ cup water and ¼ medium avocado.

1 tablespoon of lemon juice.

¾ cup frozen mango.

1/4 cup frozen raspberries.

1 tablespoon of agave (optional).

Directions:

In a blender, combine water, avocado, lemon juice, mango, raspberries, and optional agave. Blend until smooth.

Nutrition Value (per serving):

188	7g	32g	2g
Calories	Fat	Carbs	Protein

Recipes for Nutrient-Dense Smoothies

Here are some nutrient-dense smoothie recipes that are rich in vitamins, minerals, antioxidants, and fiber to promote your health and well-being:

1. For a mood boost, combine orange and turmeric.

Ingredients: Serves one.
- 1/2 cup frozen mango.
- 1/2 cup frozen pineapple chunks.
- 1 thumb of turmeric
- ½ thumb ginger
- ½ frozen banana.
- 1 tablespoon coconut butter or coconut flakes
- 2 cups orange juice.

2. For more protein, try a chocolate strawberry protein smoothie.

Ingredients: Serves one.
2 cups frozen strawberries.
1 tablespoon nut butter of your choosing.
1 scoop of chocolate protein powder of your choosing
1 cup milk of your choice
A touch of cinnamon.
Two softened dates.

3. Green Power Smoothie.

Ingredients: Serves one
1 cup spinach.
1/2 cup kale.
1/2 cucumber.
One green apple, cored and cut
1/2 avocado.
1 tablespoon of chia seeds.
1 tablespoon of hemp seeds.
1 cup almond milk or coconut water.
Juice from 1/2 lemon
Optional: 1 teaspoon of honey or maple syrup for sweetness.

4. Berry Blast Smoothie

Ingredients: Serves one.

1 cup mixed berries (such strawberries, blueberries, and raspberries)
1/2 banana.
1 tablespoon almond or peanut butter.
1 tablespoon flaxseeds or flaxmeal
1 cup spinach or kale.
1 cup almond milk or yogurt.
Optional: 1 teaspoon of honey or maple syrup for sweetness.

5. Tropical Turmeric Smoothie

Ingredients: Serves one.
1/2 cup pineapple chunks.
1/2 cup mango chunks.
1 banana.
1 teaspoon of turmeric powder.
1/2 teaspoon ginger powder (or raw ginger)
1 tablespoon of coconut oil.
1 cup almond milk or coconut water.
Optional: One tablespoon of honey or maple syrup for sweetness.

Instructions:

1. Combine all of the ingredients in a blender.
2. Blend until smooth and creamy.
3. Add additional honey, maple syrup, or liquid to get the desired sweetness or consistency.
4. Pour into a glass and drink immediately.

Incorporating Somatic Principles into Nutrition

We frequently approach nutrition through the prism of macronutrients, calories, and attaining particular goals such as weight loss or muscle building. While these factors are essential, a genuinely holistic approach to eating takes into account the deeper relationship between what we eat and how it impacts our bodies and minds. This is where somatic principles come in handy, directing us toward a more conscious and embodied approach to self-care.

Somatics Reveals the Hidden Language of Food:

- Somatic activities emphasize interoception, or the capacity to detect internal cues such as hunger, fullness, and bodily feelings. Tuning into these subtle cues allows us to have a better grasp of how food affects us beyond bodily reactions. Here's how.
- Body awareness: Pay attention to your body's sensations after consuming various meals. Does a specific meal make you feel invigorated or sluggish? Which textures or tastes cause cravings or discomfort?
- Emotional connection: Consider your emotional ties with eating. Do you use food to soothe, celebrate, or numb your emotions? Are there certain foods that elicit emotional responses?
- Mindful Eating: Slow down, chew each bite, and take in the flavor, texture, and scent of your food. This mindful approach encourages deliberate decisions and gratitude for the nutrients you provide your body.

Somatic Principles for a Nourishing Journey.

Intuitive Eating: Rather than following strict diets, practice intuitive eating by listening to your body's hunger and fullness cues. Learn to discriminate between genuine hunger and emotional desires.

Mindful Movement: Before or after meals, use mild movement routines such as yoga or tai chi to improve digestion and body awareness.

thankfulness and Presence: Practice thankfulness for both the food you eat and the act of replenishing oneself. Be present in the moment, focused on the eating experience rather than distractions.

Explore Food as Information: View food as more than simply calories; it is information that effects your body's processes. Listen to how different meals make you feel and make your choices appropriately.

Connection to Source: Think about the origin and ethical implications of your dietary choices. Connecting with local farmers, learning about food production, and thoughtful meal preparation may all help you appreciate it more.

Advantages of the Somatic Approach to Nutrition:
1. Improved Digestive Health: Listening to your body's signals can help you discover foods that cause digestive problems and make educated decisions for better gut health.
2. Reduced Emotional Eating: By recognizing the emotional link to food, you may break bad habits and eat more intuitively in response to your body's requirements.
3. Enhanced Body Image: Somatic awareness encourages a greater appreciation for your body and its specific requirements, shifting the emphasis away from restricting standards.
4. Greater Food Satisfaction: Mindfulness and mindfulness during meals can boost enjoyment and satisfaction while decreasing cravings and overeating.
5. Holistic Well-Being: Nurturing oneself via mindful food and activity routines promotes a well-rounded approach to physical and mental health.

Supporting Weight Loss with Healthy Eating

Nicole was a woman who had struggled with her weight for many years. Despite attempting a variety of diets and fitness regimes, she was always left feeling dissatisfied and dejected. Nicole, determined to make a long-term difference, decided to try a different strategy.

She began by educating herself on nutrition and the value of balanced meals. Nicole learnt how to eat healthily by concentrating on entire foods such as fruits, vegetables, lean meats, and whole grains. She also realized the need of portion management, learning to listen to her body's hunger and fullness cues. Nicole integrated weight reduction smoothies into her daily routine, following recipes from a book that offered nutrient-dense alternatives to help her achieve her objectives. These smoothies satiated her desires while also providing her with necessary nutrition and energy for the day.

Nicole started doing somatic exercises from this book in addition to her healthier eating habits. These exercises helped her become more aware of her body, improve her posture, and relieve stress that had previously hampered her weight reduction attempts. Nicole experienced physical and emotional improvements as her trip progressed. Her clothes started to fit better, she had more energy during the day, and she felt more comfortable in her own self. Nicole's friends and family saw her transformation and were encouraged by her devotion and success.

Nicole eventually achieved her weight reduction objectives while also developing a healthy connection with food and her body. She understood that long-term weight loss required more than just sticking to a diet or following a tight exercise regimen—it was about adopting long-term lifestyle adjustments that improved her entire health.

Nicole's experience demonstrates that with perseverance, education, and the correct tools, anybody can reach their health and weight reduction objectives. Her path demonstrates the power of nutritious nutrition, mindful activity, and tenacity in generating long-term transformation.

Incorporating healthy eating habits is essential for supporting weight loss goals. By focusing on nutrient-dense foods, portion control, and mindful eating practices, you can create a sustainable approach to weight management. Here are key principles to consider:

- Balanced and Nutrient-Dense Diet: Aim for a balanced diet that includes an array of nutrient-dense foods such as fruits, vegetables, whole grains, lean proteins, and healthy fats. These meals give important nutrients while also leaving you feeling satiated and invigorated.
- Meal Control: Be cautious of your meal proportions to avoid overeating. Use smaller plates, bowls, and utensils to help manage quantities, and listen to your body's hunger and fullness cues.
- Mindful Eating: Stay present throughout meals, relish each mouthful, and pay attention to your body's hunger and fullness cues. Avoid screens and multitasking while eating.
- Hydration: Drink lots of water throughout the day. Thirst may sometimes be confused for hunger, so staying hydrated might help you avoid unneeded snacks.
- Nutritious Snacking: To satiate hunger between meals, select nutritious snacks such as fruits, vegetables, almonds, or yogurt. Avoid manufactured snacks that are heavy in sugar, salt, and harmful fats.
- Limiting Processed Foods and Sugary Drinks: Cut your intake of processed foods, sugary snacks, and beverages high in added sugars. These foods can cause weight gain and may lack necessary nutrients.
- Meal Planning and Preparation: Plan out your meals ahead of time to ensure they are balanced and nutritious. This can help you make healthier decisions and prevent impulsive, harmful choices.
- Regular Physical Activity: Combine healthy eating with regular physical activity to support weight loss. Somatic exercises, such as those in your book, may be an important part of your workout program, helping to increase body awareness, movement efficiency, and general well-being.

Weight Loss Smoothies

My book includes weight loss smoothie recipes that can be a handy and nutritious way to promote weight reduction. These smoothies are intended to be nutrient-dense, with ingredients that induce satiety, supply important nutrients, and aid in metabolism. They can be used as meal substitutes or snacks, depending on your dietary requirements and preferences.

Somatic Exercises for Weight Loss

In addition to healthy eating and weight loss smoothies, my book offers somatic exercises that are particularly designed to promote weight reduction objectives. These exercises are designed to improve body awareness, increase movement efficiency, and reduce tension in the body, all of which can help to general well-being and a healthy weight.

Conclusion

Congratulations on finishing "Somatic Exercises for Beginners: Weight Loss," a complete guide to enhancing your health and well-being through mindful exercise and nutritious nutrition. Throughout this book, you've learned useful ideas and techniques to help you with your weight reduction journey and beyond. Let's go over some major elements and provide advice for long-term success:

Recap of Key Points:

Somatic Exercises: Somatic exercises focus on improving body awareness, releasing tension, and enhancing movement efficiency. Regular somatic exercise can help you improve your posture, flexibility, and general health.

Healthy Eating: A well-balanced, nutrient-dense diet can help you lose weight. Whole foods, portion management, and mindful eating practices can help you make long-term improvements to your eating habits.

Weight Loss Smoothies: The weight loss smoothie recipes in this book are nutritious, easy to prepare, and may be a tasty addition to your daily diet. These smoothies are intended to deliver critical nutrients while also helping you achieve your weight loss objectives.

Mindful Living: Mindfulness is essential for long-term success. By being observant of your food habits, exercise regimen, and general lifestyle choices, you can make informed decisions that benefit your health and well-being.

Tips for Beginners:

Start Slow: If you're new to somatic workouts or healthy eating, set tiny, attainable objectives. Gradually increase your practice and make small improvements to your diet.

Listen to your body. Pay attention to your body's cues for hunger, fullness, and exhaustion. Respect your body's boundaries and don't push yourself too hard too quickly.

Be patient: Weight reduction and lifestyle improvements need time. Instead of striving for perfection, focus on making progress and celebrating minor triumphs.

Stay Consistent: Consistency is essential for seeing outcomes. Incorporate somatic workouts and good eating habits into your everyday routine to make them a permanent part of your life.

Motivation for Long-Term Success:

As you continue your journey with somatic workouts and healthy eating, keep in mind that success is more than simply achieving a certain weight or appearance; it's about feeling good in your body, increasing your overall health, and cultivating a positive connection with food and movement. Accept the process, be gentle to yourself, and remain dedicated to your well-being. With commitment and effort, you may reach your weight reduction objectives and live a healthier, happier life. Keep up the wonderful effort, and best wishes for more success!

I Have a Request

Dear Readers,

I hope you've found "Somatic Exercises for Beginners: Weight Loss" to be a valuable resource on your journey to improved health and well-being. Your feedback is incredibly important to me as an author, and I would greatly appreciate it if you could take a moment to leave a review of the book on Amazon. Your honest review will not only help other readers discover the book but also provide me with valuable insights to improve future editions.

Additionally, I invite you to follow my Author Central page https://www.amazon.com/author/drkamakamzy.com to stay updated on new releases, special offers, and exclusive content. By following my page, you'll be among the first to know about any updates or additions to the book and have the opportunity to engage with me directly.

Thank you for your support and for being a part of this journey. I look forward to hearing your thoughts and continuing to provide you with valuable resources for your health and wellness.

Warm regards,

Dr. Kama Kamzy

ADDITIONAL RESOURCES

Explore more books by Dr. Kama Kamzy that cover a range of topics related to health, wellness, and mindful living:

Managing Blood Pressure Through Exercise: Unlocking the Path to Lifelong Cardiovascular Wellness: The Natural and Effective Step to Lower or Manage Your Blood Pressure Without Prescription Drugs.

ULTIMATE YOGA GUIDE FOR HEART HEALTH: Unlocking the Healing Power of Yoga: A Comprehensive Guide with Pictorial Postures and Heart-Healthy Diets for … Your Mind, and Elevating Your Well-Being.

You can find these books and more on Amazon. Stay updated on new releases and exclusive content by following Dr. Kama Kamzy Author Central page https://www.amazon.com/author/drkamakamzy.com

Thank you for your interest in my work, and I hope these resources continue to inspire and support your journey to holistic well-being.

Warm regards.